Advanced Practice in Nursing

Under the Auspices of the International Council of Nurses (ICN)

Series Editor
Christophe Debout, GIP-IFITS
Health Chair Sciences- Po Paris/IDS UMR Inserm 1145
Paris, France

This series of concise monographs, endorsed by the International Council of Nurses, explores various aspects of advanced practice nursing at the international level.

The ICN International Nurse Practitioner/Advanced Practice Nursing Network definition has been adopted for this series to define advanced practice nursing: "A Nurse Practitioner/Advanced Practice Nurse is a registered nurse who has acquired the expert knowledge base, complex decision-making skills and clinical competencies for expanded practice, the characteristics of which are shaped by the context and/or country in which s/he is credentialed to practice. A master's degree is recommended for entry level."

At the international level, advanced practice nursing encompasses two professional profiles:

Nurse practitioners (NPs) who have mastered advanced practice nursing, and are capable of diagnosing, making prescriptions for and referring patients. Though they mainly work in the community, some also work in hospitals. Clinical nurse specialists (CNSs) are expert nurses who deliver high-quality nursing care to patients and promote quality care and performance in nursing teams.

The duties performed by these two categories of advanced practice nurses on an everyday basis can be divided into five interrelated roles:

Clinical practice
Consultation
Education
Leadership
Research

The series addresses four topics directly related to advanced practice nursing:

APN in practice (NPs and CNSs)
Education and continuous professional development for advanced practice nurses
Managerial issues related to advanced practice nursing
Policy and regulation of advanced practice nursing

The contributing authors are mainly APNs (NPs and CNSs) recruited from the ICN International Nurse Practitioner/Advanced Practice Nursing Network. They include clinicians, educators, researchers, regulators and managers, and are recognized as experts in their respective fields.

Each book within the series reflects the fundamentals of nursing / advanced practice nursing and will promote evidence-based nursing.

More information about this series at https://link.springer.com/bookseries/13871

Maria Kidner

Successful Advanced Practice Nurse Role Transition

A Structured Process to Developing Professional Identity through Role Transition

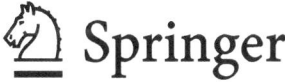 Springer

Maria Kidner
LEAP Leadership
Lander, WY, USA

ISSN 2511-3917   ISSN 2511-3925   (electronic)
Advanced Practice in Nursing
ISBN 978-3-030-53001-3   ISBN 978-3-030-53002-0   (eBook)
https://doi.org/10.1007/978-3-030-53002-0

This Springer imprint is published by the registered company Springer Nature Switzerland AG
The registered company address is: Gewerbestrasse 11, 6330 Cham, Switzerland

Preface

The development of this book came about from an opportunity and honor to work on the preparation for the new Advanced Practice Nurse (APN) role for the Kingdom of Bahrain in 2018. As I pondered the path of becoming an advanced practice nurse and the process of role transition, I recognized that many nurses expanding their education to the APN level are already strong nurses yet are anxious about the new role of APN. This increased APN role transition stress is often related to the increased accountability, responsibility, and authority required upon entering the APN practice. Thus, understanding APN role transition, finding a deeper understanding of who one is as an APN, becoming attached to the profession of APN, and developing the skills of each aspect of the APN role became the focus of this book. From 2014 to 2019 I developed a process which nurses can gain an understanding about self and working relationships. This process grew from my work in Guyana, South America and Rwanda, Africa. It is called the LEAP Process, which stands for "Leadership, Engagement, Accountability, and Professionalism." As I wove the topics of role transition and leadership together, I recognized there needs to be an enhanced understanding of our self-concept and professional identity as APN to improve successful APN role transition. Topics of self-concept, self-efficacy, personal identity, professional identity, and role transition are often not included in formal APN education. I wanted to write a book that would provide APNs the steps to build the skills needed for a successful APN role transition. It is the concepts and process of becoming our best that I want to share with all APN students, faculty, and nurses.

This book was written to guide APN students through their role transition from a generalist nurse to the APN role. To successfully accomplish this APN role transitional process, students need to understand first there is an evidence-based process which students experience role transition; and second there are skills and activities that can aid in the development of one's professional identity, build a positive self-concept, and role transition with less stress.

Self-reflection is key to help APN students to review their self-concept while gaining an understanding about their potential influences on being an advanced practice nurse, leading teams, and making changes. Understanding oneself helps a person to embrace their chosen professional role to be strong during times of push-back, confusion, and poor support. I have drawn on my personal nursing experiences including labor and delivery, medical-surgical hospital nursing, and as an

APN in emergency, primary care, and cardiology. My international work in Guyana, South America, Rwanda, Africa, and Vietnam has greatly enriched my nursing and ability to develop this book. My experiences within many healthcare professional organizations widened my understanding of APN influence and impact. My memberships involvement in nursing and social organizations increased my understanding of the importance of professional and community involvement. My experiences as an educator, clinical instructor, autonomous healthcare provider, and as an entrepreneur have provided me opportunities to build, present, and evaluate educational material along with partnering with students on their professional identity journeys.

Lander, WY, USA   Maria Kidner

Acknowledgments

The construction of this book, from the mist of my thoughts to written words on a page, has been a multifaceted effort over many years as I explored the adventures life placed before me. I will start my list of indebted gratitude with my father who many decades ago inspired me to look at leadership as guiding others to become their best. Next would be my mentor, Dr. Michael Zychowicz, who mentored me through a clinical strategic plan project through the American Association of Nurse Practitioners in 2009. He taught me the importance of understanding myself and recognizing my impact on others.

This book commenced after a discussion with Dr. Madrean Schober who suggested to solidify my ideas of role transition and professional identity as integral parts of pre-leadership needs. Thus, this book was born. I am deeply humbled and indebted to those who spent many hours reading and sharing their ideas, concerns, and suggestions on this book. I especially want to mention Dr. Madrean Schober, Dr. Mary Beth Stepans, and Kathy Pappas who read every word and discussed every chapter to provide mentorship and lively conversations.

This book could not have come together without the innumerable hours other nurse educators, practicing clinicians, and nurse leaders provided to me in reading, correcting, and sharing insights throughout the entire process. These include: educators Dr. Mary Burman, Dr. Kathy Wheeler, Dr. Deb Gray, Dr. Kristina Davis, Dr. Savitri Singh-Carlson, Dr. Barb Turner, and Dr. Judith Berg; nurse practitioners Mary Behrens, Alicia LePard, and Lukia DeWitt Beverly; international consultant Dr. Madrean Schober; my international colleagues Mr. Hai Ngo Thanh (Vietnam), Heather McGrath (Jamaica), Martin Nsengimana (Rwanda), Christian Ntakirutimana (Rwanda), and Bonisile Nsibandze (Eswati); and DNP students Adrienne Reddick, Kenita Murray, and Jessica Wallace. A special thanks to Dr. Hillary Barnes and the many emails we shared.

I would also like to point out the graphic artwork in this book is by graphic artist, Derek Rake, who devoted hours translating my ideas to graphic models. My deepest thanks and admiration of his work.

Lastly, yet profoundly important, is my thanks and appreciation to my husband who patiently supported me through the numerous hours I spent on the computer, reading literature, and taking notes as we travelled and at home. I often had my computer and headset on while in the car, in hotels, at family events, and at home. Martin knew when to let me type and when to pull me a way for a needed break or when to lift my head to witness a grand sunset, or majestic scenery as we travelled. Thank you, everyone for guiding and supporting me through the wonderful and detailed experience of writing a book for APNs. I am honored.

About This Book

Message to Readers

It is my intent to find ways to inspire you to be curious about the topics presented in this book. I want to provide you with ideas about forming your opinions and thoughts with subsequent paths for you to follow to develop your personal strengths, values, vision, and mission. Building upon your personal ideas, you will then expand how you encounter others as an APN clinical leader (both formal and informal) with your social influences building on the enhanced responsibility, accountability, and authority of an APN.

I have read many books on leadership and a common process is to tell the reader "what" they should obtain or do ("you should have your own values" or "you should build capacity of others"). Yet many books do not tell you how to gain the skill! I have designed this book to help you find the skills needed for your successful APN role transition. To accomplish this, I have provided you many activities and ample space to write your thoughts, plans, and ideas. In the simple act of writing, you will greatly increase your chance of success.

I recognize the amount of time it will take to answer every question. By writing your thoughts you will increase your ability to become a stronger, wiser clinician and leader. Please write, doodle, draw pictures, make comments, and use this book as much as your creative heart inspires you to do as you become who you are meant to be. Then keep this book in your bookcase and every year open it and review your words to keep your plans active along with gaining knowledge of your growth from novice to expert. Should you want to share your journey of role transitions with me, please feel free to contact me.

Dr. Maria Kidner
Maria.kidner@leapleadership.org
This book provides you with insights concerning:

- The APN role and scope of practice.
- The importance of understanding your country's laws and regulations concerning the APN role.
- The common processes of APN role transition through a concept analysis.

- How to be introspective with forethought concerning yourself and developing a map for your future through personal strategic planning.
- An enhanced understanding possible relationships and communication barriers an APN can experience.
- Multiple activities to develop a strong and healthy identity of who you are as an APN.

Ultimately, your role as an APN is to provide high-quality, evidence-based patient or community care to impact the health and well-being of your community. That care is deeply embedded in who you are as person, as nurse, and as APN. Your values, attitudes, behaviors, and beliefs make up your perceived identity of professional self as APN and the APN profession within your country and the world (Lombarts et al. 2014). Plus, your attitudes and behaviors are impacted by your workplace organizational structure, culture, teamwork, motivational support (leadership), and the professional patient interactions of physicians, APNs, and nursing (Lombarts et al. 2014).

APNs are needed worldwide. The APN role enhances healthcare of populations worldwide. The process of role and scope of practice change from a generalist nurse to an APN can be a complex and challenging process. The common emotions of self-doubt, confusion, isolation, role ambiguity, and fear (Barnes 2015; Faraz 2016 Hussein et al. 2017; Owens 2019) can be mitigated through graining and understanding of the common APN role transition process and developing strategies to build one's self-concept, self-efficacy, and professional identity (Barnes 2015; Goliroshan et al. 2021; Owens 2019).

You are on a challenging educational journey that comprises curiosity to seek new information, courage to complete a successful role transition to APN and to become a change agent and support to your patients and nursing. You have the dedication and ability to work hard, the perseverance to overcome barriers, the understanding who you are through your self-concept, self-efficacy, and professional identity. You have the tools of a personal transition plan to guide your progress. Now it is up to you to recognize your supportive stakeholders, become a mentee, and fully understand your strengths and wisdom you have gained. Congratulations on your APN graduate education progress.

References

Barnes H (2015) Exploring the factors that influence nurse practitioner role transition. J Nurse Pract 11(2):178–183. https://doi.org/10.1016/j.nurpra.2014.11.004

Faraz A (2016) Novice nurse practitioner workforce transition into primary care: a literature review. West J Nurs Res 38(11);1531–1545. https://doi.org/10.177/0193945916649587

Goliroshan S, Nobahar M, Raeisdana N, Ebadinejad Z, Aziznejadroshan P (2021) The protective role of professional self-concept and job embeddedness on nurses' burnout: structural equation modeling. BMC Nursing 20;203. https://doi.org/10.1186/s12912-021-00727-8

Hussein R, Everett B, Ramjan LM, Hu W, Salamonson Y (2017) New graduate nurses' experiences in a clinical specialty: a follow up study of newcomer perceptions of transitional support. BMC Nurs 16:42. https://doi.org/10.1186/s12912-017-0236-0. PMID: 28775671; PMCID: PMC5534089

Lombarts KMJMH, Plochg T, Thompson CA (2014) Arah OA on behalf of the DUQuE project consortium. Measuring professionalism in medicine and nursing: results of a european survey. PloS ONE 9(5):e97069. https://doi.org/10.1371/journal.pone.0097069

Owens R (2019) Nurse practitioner role transition and identity development in rural health care settings: a scoping review. Nursing Education Perspectives 40(3):157–161. https://doi.org/10.1097/01.NEP.0000000000000455

Contents

APN Role Transition Introduction

1

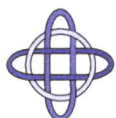

If you are reading this book, you are most likely a student studying advanced practice nursing and looking forward to a new role in nursing that has expanded responsibility, accountability, and authority to implement advanced clinical competence in providing healthcare. Or, perhaps, you are starting your first job as advanced practice nurse (APN). It is an exciting time. Yet, there is often confusion over the role of the APN. This confusion can be within yourself, from your family and friends, your fellow nurses, your patients, and even current healthcare providers due to a lack of understanding about the APN role and scope of practice. This lack of knowledge is more acute when the APN role is newly introduced into the healthcare system. If you are confused or uncertain about your ability to proceed, you are not alone as most APN students will experience feelings of uncertainty during the graduate education. This book is designed to help you understand APN role transition and provide steps for your future success.

This chapter introduces a structured process of developing a professional identity and nursing role transition from a generalist nurse to an APN. Throughout this book you will learn processes to help you understand the expanded nursing responsibility and the potential outcomes with implementation of the advanced practice role. This chapter provides answers to a series of questions concerning the APN role and offers definitions to be applied in this book.

The APN is an exciting role for nurses to seize an active position in improving patient outcomes, support nursing, and advocate for others. It is a role that requires the APN to maintain integrity to the role and scope of practice in order to build trust with all stakeholders involved.

© The Author(s), under exclusive license to Springer Nature Switzerland AG 2022
M. Kidner, *Successful Advanced Practice Nurse Role Transition*, Advanced
Practice in Nursing, https://doi.org/10.1007/978-3-030-53002-0_1

Exemplar-CNS

Allison has recently graduated with her master's degree and obtained her license as an APN-Clinical Nurse Specialist. She has taken a new role as CNS in her hospital where she previously had been employed as a nurse for 7 years. She will be one of the first APNs in her hospital. Allison learned about the role transition process during her graduate education and decided to use that information to guide this phase of her transition into APN practice. As soon as she learned about the importance of a mentorship, she reached out to both her floor supervisor and the director of nursing who welcomed the mentorship process. In addition, she has worked hard to maintain her friendships and working relationships where she will go from coworker to APN. She provided information about her CNS role and scope of practice to her nursing colleagues as she went through her education and clinical practicum. Allison is eager to start her new role and is confident that she can successfully transition her role from generalist nurse to CNS.

Exemplar-NP

Kelly has graduated with his master's degree and obtained his license as an APN-Nurse Practitioner. He is returning to the city where his family lives to join a local primary care clinic. He has not returned home since starting his APN graduate education. Kelly is anxious about returning home, starting a new nursing role, and joining a practice in which he has little experience as a primary care provider. He discussed his concerns of lack of confidence and fears in being the first NP in his clinic with a trusted nursing professor. Together they developed a plan to provide support and mentorship via the internet to help guide Kelly's transition into practice.

1.1   Definitions

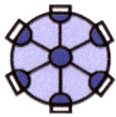

Professional identity Your professional identity is your self-concept of who you are within your profession and how you uphold the attributes, values, and image of that profession (Fitzgerald 2020).

Role   A *role* describes a related set of activities and expected behavior patterns, determined by the individual's function in society, that the person performs to complete a process, or series of actions (Owens 2019).

Role Transition   Role transition is the process in which a person, through a series of events, disengages from one role and engages in another role using energy, resiliency, and personal dedication (Barnes 2015; Holt 2008; Moran and Nairn 2018).

Structured process   A process that is based in evidence, planned, thoughtful, and executed according to the plan is structured. There is a start event, a series of tasks/events, and a subsequent end event. The goal of an educational structured process is to support students to grow as individuals, gain confidence, and success (Berke 2018; Kidner 2019). When it is applied within this book, a structured process concerns APN role transition.

1.2   What Is Role Transition?

The APN role transition process is characterized by disconnectedness and unfamiliar expectations (Barnes 2015; Faraz 2016; Holt 2008; Moran and Nairn 2018; Reynolds and Mortimer 2021). Role transitions occur throughout our lives in many domains including occupation, employment, physical health, and even relationship changes. A role transition includes a personal identity change that occurs through the embodiment of new knowledge, skills, role relationships, and role expectations (Owens 2019).

APN role transition is the process a nurse experiences starting with the decision to become an APN and continues through the graduate educational process into the first year of the APN job. In the first APN job, the new APN must disengage from the previous role as a generalist nurse and assimilate the enhanced responsibility, accountability, and scope of practice of the APN into the new APN job (Barnes 2015; Owens 2019; Rasmussen et al. 2018). That experience is role transition. Your decision to become an APN began your role transition process.

Role transition is considered a *macro* transition if it is from a generalist nurse to an advanced practice nurse. Role transition is considered a *micro* transition if it is from the role of the nurse advocate to the role of a formal nurse leader (Smith et al. 2019). Yet, role transitions no matter how simple or complex are enhanced with a structured (planned and thoughtful) process for successful transition. Understanding the process will help internalize the transition and understand the emotions involved while gaining the knowledge and skills required for the new role. Role transition is a process.

Role transition is an individual process that transcends APN role development. Each nurse who chooses to expand their knowledge to develop from a generalist or specialized nurse to an APN will experience a variety of emotions as they transition from one nursing role to another. This role transition involves personal, professional, intellectual, emotional, skill, and relationship changes that occur in a relatively predictable path (Barnes 2015; Duchscher 2008). If a person understands there is a predictable process for a successful role transition and executes a plan to experience the role transition process, then it will be a *structured role transition* (Barnes 2015; Alshawush et al. 2020).

The stress of graduate education, working, family obligations, and role transition will mix with the excitement and curiosity of the upcoming future (Barnes 2015; Duchscher 2008). It is important to understand that the experience of APN role transition is highly individualized, yet common themes are present. To provide you with steps for successful structured role transition, the 2015 Barnes concept analysis of role transition has been chosen (Barnes 2015).

1.3   What Is Professional Identity?

A professional identity is a personalized self-concept of how you fit into a professional role with your values, ethics, knowledge, and skills within the context of a particular profession that is obtained through the socialization process of formal education, clinical practice, and workplace experiences (Haghighat et al. 2020; Owens 2019). Within your role transition from a generalist nurse to an APN, your professional identity will expand from that of your current nursing role to include your increased knowledge, skills, and critical thinking associated with the APN. Simply put your professional identity is your perception of what it means to act and to be an APN (Rasmussen et al. 2018).

To gain a professional identity requires self-introspection and comparison of your personal values and attitudes to what you learn as you go through your educational process in relation to the reality of the workplace culture and expected role attributes (Hunter and Cook 2018). Through mentoring, observing other APNs, building trust relationships, and developing friendships you can establish a professional identity that will provide you a foundation in which you can develop your APN career.

1.4   What Is the APN Role All About?

The APN role is the nursing response to provide unmet healthcare needs of people. To gain an understanding of the APN role, one must understand the definitions of nursing and types of APNs recognized internationally.

1.4.1   Nursing and APN Role Definitions

The act of caring for others is as old as the human race. There has been an intuitive response in providing comfort and assurance to those who were sick. Over the centuries people gained knowledge and skills through both informal and formal processes which became nursing roles. Recently, the advanced nursing roles developed through societal needs, governmental support, and nursing capabilities. Each country has developed their own definitions, titles, scope of practice, and requirements. Internationally, there were similarities in role definitions, scope of practice, and educational processes. Yet, the inconsistencies increase the difficulties in understanding the implementation process, society acceptance, and potential impacts. Thus, it is important to start this book with commonly accepted definitions based on a review of the literature and available resources.

Definition of Nursing   As nursing has developed in each country, the understanding of nursing and the specific definition of nursing has varied. As nursing roles expand, it is important to understand the true essence of nursing. The definition of "Nursing" can be culture and country dependent. It can also be difficult to find a well-documented definition of "Nursing." Below are a few examples found:

International Council of Nursing (ICN) (2020)
Nursing encompasses autonomous and collaborative care of individuals of all ages, families, groups and communities, sick or well and in all settings. Nursing includes the promotion of health, prevention of illness, and the care of ill, disabled and dying people. Advocacy, promotion of a safe environment, research, participation in shaping health policy and in patient and health systems management, and education are also key nursing roles (ICN 2020) (https://www.icn.ch/nursing-policy/nursing-definitions#:~:text=Definition%20of%20a%20Nurse,nursing%20in%20his%2Fher%20country. Accessed 5/2/2021).

World Health Organization
Nursing encompasses autonomous and collaborative care of individuals of all ages, families, groups and communities, sick or well and in all settings. It includes the promotion of health, the prevention of illness, and the care of ill, disabled and dying people. Nurses play a critical role in healthcare and are often the unsung heroes in healthcare facilities and emergency response. They are often the first to detect health emergencies and work on the front lines of disease prevention and the delivery of primary healthcare, including promotion, prevention, treatment and rehabilitation (https://www.who.int/health-topics/nursing#tab=tab_1 access 26 April 2022).

Florence Nightingale
Florence Nightingale's Environmental Theory defined Nursing as "the act of utilizing the patient's environment to assist him in his recovery" (https://www.onwardhealthcare.com/resources/blog/nursing-news/florence-nightingale/ accessed 26 April 26, 2022).

China (2004)
The definition for "Nursing" in China changes in the translation to English because the original language is rooted in Chinese medicine and eastern ideologies that cannot be translated. The translated definition is:

> Nursing means to understand the dynamic health status of a person, to dialectically verify health concerns, and to devise interventions with the goal of assisting the person to master the appropriate health knowledge and skills for the attainment of optimal well-being (Pang et al. 2004).

Royal College of Nursing, England (2002)

Nursing is the use of clinical judgment and the provision of care to enable people to promote, improve, maintain, or recover health or, when death is inevitable, to die peacefully (Scott 2002).

United States of America (2010)

In 2010 the American Nurses Association defined nursing as: "the protection, promotion, and optimization of health and abilities; prevention of illnesses and injury; alleviation of suffering through the diagnosis and treatment of human response; and advocacy in the care of individuals, families, communities, and populations" (Blair 2019, p. 32).

Nursing Role Definitions

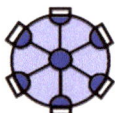

A nurse The nurse is a person who has completed a program of basic, generalized nursing education and is authorized by the appropriate regulatory authority to practice nursing in his/her country. This includes generalist nurses, specialist nurses, nurse educators, nurses with master's or PhD degrees, nurses in formal leadership roles, and APNs (https://www.icn.ch/nursing-policy/nursing-definitions#:~:text=Definition%20of%20a%20Nurse,nursing%20in%20his%2Fher%20country. Accessed 5/2/2021).

A "**generalist nurse**" is a nurse who has completed their country's required education and can provide nursing care to patients in diverse settings following the plans of an APN and/or physician. A generalist nurse is considered to be a professional capable of developing care at any point in the healthcare systems and settings. Therefore, the nursing education must encompass knowledge, skills, and attitudes that enable the student to develop competences for the comprehensive care of the patients from birth to death in all settings (Massaroli et al. 2019).

A "*specialized nurse*" The specialized nurse is a generalist nurse who has obtained additional knowledge via on-the-job education, short courses, or workshops in a specific disease process (such as cardiology, oncology, or wound management) or acute care unit (such as neonatology, emergency room, or surgery) or population focus (such as pediatrics or geriatrics) (Tracy and O'Grady 2019). A specialized nurse is valued in healthcare systems and can provide care for complex health issues within their increased knowledge area within a defined scope of practice (Halm 2021; ICN 2020). A specialized nurse can progress to the role of CNS/APN as countries develop the graduate APN educational process, legal recognition, and regulations (ICN 2020).

An "Advanced Practice Nurse" (APN) An APN is a generalist or specialized nurse who has completed a graduate education program that is specific to advanced practice nursing and has been authorized to practice as an APN. The 2020 ICN Guidelines on Advanced Practice Nursing states: "An APN is one who has acquired, through additional education, the expert knowledge base, complex decision-making skills and clinical competencies for expanded nursing practice, the characteristics of which are shaped by the context in which they are credential to practice" (ICN 2020, p. 9).

The ICN Guidelines on Advanced Practice Nursing clearly identifies the advanced educational requirement of the APN as a graduate (masters or doctorate) education. Yet, the APN education and philosophy is based upon nursing, nursing principles, and nursing theories (ICN 2020).

Under the APN title, three common APN roles are:

1. Clinical Nurse Specialist
2. Nurse Practitioner
3. Nurse Anesthetist

- Note: Internationally the Nurse Midwife (NM) role can be a layperson, an undergraduate nursing degree, or a non-nursing health professional. The wide variety of people providing care through the midwife role can create confusion when discussing academic preparation and scope of practice. For midwives who are also nurses their scope of practice and academic preparation will determine whether they can be identified as APN in a healthcare system.
- Therefore, the NM role is not included in the current 2020 ICN APN definition because not all NM are APN, yet those who have APN graduate education in NM can be an APN.

Clinical Nurse Specialist (CNS) The CNS is an APN with a minimum of a master's degree with enhanced education and clinical practicums focused on a specialized area of nursing practice that impacts systems, outcomes, and patient care (ICN 2020). The CNS provides direct patient care and indirect care that influences the care and outcomes of patients (as nurse consultant, clinical leadership, develops, plans and directs programs of care) (ICN 2020). This advanced specialized expertise may be defined by:

- Population (such as pediatrics, geriatrics, or women's health)
- Setting (such as critical care or emergency room)
- Disease or medical subspecialty (such as diabetes or oncology)
- Type of care (such as psychiatric or rehabilitation)
- Type of problem (such as pain, wounds, or stress)
  (https://nacns.org/about-us/what-is-a-cns/ accessed 4.30/2021)

Nurse Practitioner (NP) The NP is an APN with a minimum of a master's degree combined with extensive clinical education who can provide healthcare across the lifespan autonomously and in coordination with other healthcare professionals. The graduate education is specifically designed to educate NPs to assess, diagnose, treat, and manage both chronic and acute illnesses in both inpatient and outpatient community settings. In addition, NPs can order, supervise, conduct, and interpret diagnostic and laboratory tests (ICN 2020; AANP 2015). In some countries, the NP has the authority to write and manage prescription medications autonomously. A unique aspect of NP practice is the emphasis on the health and well-being of the whole person with health promotion and lifestyle management as the cornerstone of the care provided.

Nurse Anesthetist (NA) The NA is an APN who has completed a master's degree (or higher) educational program specific to anesthesia and who has the knowledge, skills, and competencies to provide individualized care in anesthesia, pain management, and related anesthesia services to patients across the lifespan (International Council of Nurses Guidelines on Advanced Practice Nursing Nurse Anesthetists 2020).

1.4.2 APN's Providing Healthcare

Responding to the shortages of healthcare providers, nurses recognized the potential of providing patient-centered care focused on health, wellness, and prevention of illness would impact communities where shortages persisted (Maier et al. 2016). Yet, the APN role does not simply meet the unmet society needs of providing healthcare, the APN role is the potential of nursing to provide, support, educate, and lead others (patients and communities) to improved wellness from individuals to public health. The APN nurse practitioner, clinical nurse specialist, and nurse anesthetist roles were designed to educate nurses to provide advanced nursing healthcare services in multiple locations. Internationally these roles are implemented differently in response to the country's healthcare culture, health needs, and practice settings embracing the APN role. In general, the NP role is a direct prescriber of care to patients as a healthcare provider, and the CNS role provides quality improvement, assesses systems management, directs staff education and offers mentorship. Each role dramatically impacts the health and well-being of the persons and populations for whom they care. Both the NP and CNS may provide care in a variety of locations such as acute care hospitals, primary care and specialty care ambulatory clinics, long-term care facilities, community agencies, and in homes. In some countries, the APN is a combination of both the NP and CNS roles.

Advanced Practice Nursing should not be confused a nurse providing "medical care." APNs are nurses providing advanced nursing care using nursing paradigms and theories. Three nursing paradigms often applied to the APN role include the (1) biopsychosocial, (2) totality, and (3) simultaneity.

- A unique aspect of the biopsychosocial nursing paradigm is the assessment of both actual and potential alterations of the health continuum with subsequent patient/family education, and support for the development of healthy lifestyle strategies in addition to medicines, or medical procedures, required for that specific disease process (Borrell-Carrió et al. 2004). The two major nursing paradigms of totality and simultaneity underscore the nursing philosophy that is the foundation of APNs providing healthcare autonomously and directly to patients.

- The totality paradigm views the human–universe relationship as cause-effect in nature person as an integration of biological, psychological, sociocultural, and spiritual dimensions and considers that he or she adapts to changes in the external environment and subjectively experiences wellness and illness as a continuum of health states (Doucet and Merlin 2014; Parse 2000; Younas 2020).
- The simultaneity paradigm is embedded in a view of the human–universe relationship as a mutual process where human beings as whole entities are recognized through patterns and considered to be in continuous and simultaneous interaction with their environment (Parse 2000; Younas 2020).

APNs continue this vital nursing function of providing direct patient care and education based on nursing philosophy. Research has shown that the APN can provide high-quality, safe, and effective care internationally in most primary care visits (Maier et al. 2016; Newhouse et al. 2011; Poghosyan et al. 2017; Woo et al. 2017). A list of research supporting APN practice is provided at the end of the chapter in Appendix.

A review of international literature concerning APNs reveals multiple APN roles or levels that were described and attributed to APN practice. For the purposes of this book, the three most common roles of the APN will be utilized.

Currently, there are over 70 countries that have, or are developing, the APN role to respond to their societal needs for high-quality healthcare with improved outcomes (Bryant-Lukosius and Martin-Misener 2016). The development and integration of the APN roles has been a slow and challenging process requiring education, competency enhancements, legislation, and regulation activities on the local and national levels within each country (Bryant-Lukosius and Martin-Misener 2016; ICN 2020).

- Resource Links for review of APN development in several countries
- https://www.icn.ch/system/files/documents/2020-04/ICN_APN%20 Report_EN_WEB.pdf
- https://international.aanp.org/Content/docs/MappingOfAdvPracNursing-Competencies.pdf

1.4.3 Why Should I Become an APN?

Choosing to become an APN is a personal choice. It requires the curiosity within oneself to see a potential in an expanded role of nursing combined with the desire to progress in your professional career path. Becoming an APN requires a high sense of self-awareness that will influence your behavior and impact the quality of performance in providing healthcare to others (Dumphy et al. 2019). There are many aspects that may impact your decision to become an APN. The status of the APN role in your country will impact your need for self-competence, self-determination, and the process of successful role transition. Countries in which the APN role is successful with a consistent role definition, scope of practice, and is well known to multiple stakeholders provide support for APNs through the role transition. Other APNs can be mentors. However, even in countries where the APN role is new, every APN is expected to be strong, resilient, and able to implement role and scope of practice development. This includes promoting the APN role to multiple stakeholders, be able to negotiate multiple barriers, and develop trust relationships (Dlamini et al. 2020; Gysin et al. 2019). Ultimately, you will need to understand why you want to become an APN to facilitate your role transition.

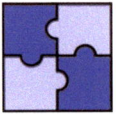

Activity List some *reasons* of why you want to become an APN

_____
_____
_____
_____
_____
_____

What can the increased accountability and responsibility of an APN include?

As a nurse you were a critical member of the healthcare team. Many nurses are responsible for developing, implementing, and evaluating the plans of care designed by a nurse, APN, physician, or other healthcare provider. However, through education and clinical practice the APN has an increased level of critical thinking and clinical competence based on advanced nursing education. This combination of enhanced critical decisions within clinical context increases the accountability, responsibility, and decision-making with enhanced authority in assessments, diagnosis, plan development, and clinical competencies of the APN. As an APN you will have increased responsibility and accountability for:

- Utilizing evidence-based pathophysiology, pharmacology, and case management knowledge
- Providing safe, effective, and high-quality direct patient care and supervising care provided by other team members
- Prescribing and monitoring evidence-based medication and treatment plans

- Being self-aware of personal limitations and making appropriate referrals to other healthcare professionals as needed
- The ability to practice autonomously
- Gaining people's trust through clinical competence and confidence
- Leading and co-coordinating care
- Managing time effectively
- Being both an informal clinical and formal leadership positions
- Having the ability and knowledge to work with change and systems
- Building workplace capacity and engagement (Darvill et al. 2018)

The level of authority through increased autonomy of the APN will vary from country to country. APNs may have increased authority to provide care by:

- Designing, prescribing, and monitoring medications of their patients
- Seeing new patients without physician supervision and diagnosing these patients
- Determining testing for a diagnosis and interpreting the results for diagnosis and subsequently developing the plan of care for that patient autonomously
- Providing healthcare in complex chronic care
- Providing healthcare in emergent situations

Perhaps a main reason you want to become an APN is because of the increased leadership opportunities. Advanced Practice Nurses are formal and informal leaders. The APN role is tied to several World Health Organization's global strategies of Human Resources for Health (HRH). Objective three of the HRH is to build the capacity of leadership on national and international levels (Bryant-Lukosius and Martin-Misener 2016). Since the APN graduate education has a core competency of leadership, APNs will impact the HRH strategies through implementation of formal and informal leadership. The APN role will allow you to impact care delivery systems, policies, and quality of care that will promote healthy outcomes in your community. The APN role is an exciting career in which you can positively impact many people.

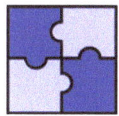

Activity List some *APN activities* of why you want to become an APN

_____
_____
_____
_____
_____
_____

1.5   How Will Gaining a Professional Identity Impact My Role Transition?

The role transition from generalized nurse to APN is often more complex than antici-pated. Unforeseen barriers from within nursing, other stakeholders, superiors, patients, and regulatory aspects can make a successful role transition difficult (Barnes 2015; Faraz 2016; Holt 2008; Moran and Nairn 2018; Reynolds and Mortimer 2021). However, taking the time to understand your personal identity as a nurse and that as an APN during your role transition is most helpful in reinforcing your confidence as APN and ability to overcome barriers implementing your APN role. Your professional and personal identities are not a single or a fixed identity but are intertwined and different within different moments or social constructs and changes with experiences and knowl-edge (Adamy et al. 2020). Your identity will give meaning to who you are as person, as a nurse, as an APN, and as a healthcare provider. Providing care to complex patients in varied locations and circumstances requires a well-developed personal paradigm of morals and ethics integrated with scientific knowledge (Haghighat et al. 2020).

This understanding of professional identity provides a foundation of trust, integ-rity, justice, and fortitude that drives APN behavior. Thus, taking the time to under-stand and work formally on your professional identity growth and development of your nursing role transition will improve your success.

1.6   How Does This Book Work?

This book is designed to supply you with knowledge and steps to understand, reflect, and achieve a successful role transition to APN through a structured process. To accomplish this, this book has been developed as a writing manual with multiple questions that will guide personal values clarification, goals setting, and identity formation along with additional activities.

The contents of the book will help you anticipate change and find the knowledge to guide you to achieve the enhanced responsibility, accountability, and authority required of an APN. Use this book as a working manual to write your answers, thoughts, and progress. The more you write, the more you will understand your own transformation from a generalist or specialist nurse to an APN.

1.7   Expected Outcomes from This APN Role Transition Book

In addition to learning what a person can do for APN role transition, this book will provide you with step-by-step instructions and guidance to obtain success-ful role transition skills. Upon completion of this book, you should be able to:

1. Gain insight through self-reflection of your personal self-concept and profes-sional identity as an APN.
2. Understand the process of role transition from a generalist nurse to an APN and gain skills to implement your personal transition process.

3. Acquire an understanding of your country and your culture's impact on your APN role.
4. Conceptualize and articulate the distinction between a generalist, non-APN specialist, and advanced practice nurse.
5. Plan, implement, and evaluate your professional role transition strategic plan.
6. Learn skills to assess, enhance, and guide your professional identity in formal, informal, and personal introspective settings.

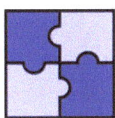

Activity Mentor qualities. Think of a nurse that you hold in high regard. What qualities do you see in that person that you admire and hope to acquire?

_____
_____
_____
_____
_____
_____
_____
_____
_____
_____
_____
_____
_____

Think about your first term in your APN graduate program. In what ways have you transitioned towards becoming an APN? How have you grown in your personal and professional life?

_____
_____
_____
_____
_____

1.8   Summary

This chapter provides you with an introduction to the topics and structure of the book. Several definitions are provided to aid in clarification including generalist nurse, specialist nurse, advanced practice nurse, clinical nurse specialist, nurse practitioner, and nurse anesthetist. The main points of this chapter include:

- The International Council of Nursing APN/NP Network is the main professional body that provides international guidelines on advanced practice nursing including the updated 2020 definition of APN. Link: https://www.icn.ch/who-we-are/icn-nurse-practitioneradvanced-practice-network-npapn-network
- Role transition from a generalist nurse to an APN is complex and individualized with the person's individual experiences, history, and philosophy impacting the process.
- An increase in the accountability, authority, and responsibility of the APN may create role transition concerns and challenges.

Appendix: References Concerning APN Quality of Care

Bauer JC (2010) Nurse practitioners as an underutilized resource for health reform: evidence-based demonstrations of cost-effectiveness. JAANP 22(4):228–231

Borgmeyer A, Gyr PM, Jamerson PA, Henry LD (2008) Evaluation of the role of the pediatric nurse practitioner in an inpatient asthma program. J Pediatr Health Care 22(5):273–281

Buerhaus P, Perloff J, Clarke S, O'Reilly-Jacob M, Zolotusky G, DesRoches CM (2018) Quality of primary care provided to medicare beneficiaries by nurse practitioners and physicians. Med Care 56(6):484–490

Carter A, Chochinov A (2007) A systematic review of the impact of nurse practitioners on cost, quality of care, satisfaction and wait times in the emergency department. Can J Emerg Med 9(4):286–295

Jackson GL, Smith VA, Edelman D, Woolson SL, Hendrix CC, Everett CM, Berkowitz TS, White BS, Morgan PA (2018) Intermediate diabetes outcomes in patients managed by physicians, nurse practitioners, or physician assistants: a cohort study. Ann Intern Med 169(12):825–835

Kippenbrock T, Emory J, Lee P, Odell E, Buron B, Morrison B (2019) A national survey of nurse practitioners' patient satisfaction outcomes. Nurs Outlook 67(6):707–712

Kleinpell RM, Grabenkort WR, Kapu AN, Constantine R, Sicoutris C (2019). Nurse practitioners and physician assistants in acute and critical care: a concise review of the literature and data 2008–2018. Crit Care Med 47(10):1442

Kurtzman ET, Barnow VS (2017) A comparison of nurse practitioners, physician assistants, and primary care physicians' patterns of practice and quality of care in health centers. Med Care 55(6):615–622

Landsperger JS, Semler MW, Wang L, Byrne DW, Wheeler AP (2016) Outcomes of nurse practitioner-developed critical care: a prospective cohort study. Chest 149(5):1146–1154

Maier CB, Aiken LH (2016) Task shifting from physicians to nurses in primary care in 39 countries: a cross-country comparative study. Eur J Public Health 26(6):927–934. https://doi.org/10.1093/eurpub/ckw098. Epub 2016 Aug 2. PMID: 27485719

Newhouse RP, Stanik-Hutt J, White KM, Johantgen M, Bass EB, Zangaro G, Wilson RF, Fountain L, Steinwachs DM, Heindel L, Weiner JP (2011) Advanced practice nurse outcomes 1990-2008: a systematic review. Nurs Econ 29(5):230–250; quiz 251. PMID: 22372080

Poghosyan L, Liu J, Norful AA (2017) Nurse practitioners as primary care providers with their own patient panels and organizational structures: a cross-sectional study. Int J Nurs Stud 74:1–7. https://doi.org/10.1016/j.ijnurstu.2017.05.004. Epub 2017 May 25. PMID: 28577459; PMCID: PMC6342506

Rantz MJ, Popejoy L, Vogelsmeier A, Galambos C, Alexander G, Flesner M, Petroski G (2018) Impact of advanced practice registered nurses on quality measures: the Missouri quality initiative experience. J Am Med Dir Assoc 19(6):541–550

Tapper EB, Hao S, Lin M, Mafi JN, McCurdy H, Parikh ND, Lok AS (2020). The quality and outcomes of care provided to patients with cirrhosis by advanced practice providers. Hepatology 71(1):225–234

Taylor A, Staruchowicz L (2012) The experience and effectiveness of nurse practitioners in orthopaedic settings: a comprehensive systematic review. JBI Libr Syst Rev 10(42 Suppl):1–22. https://doi.org/10.11124/jbisrir-2012-249. PMID: 27820153

Virani SS, Maddox TM, Chan PS, Tang F, Akeroyd JM, Risch SA, Petersen LA (2015) Provider type and quality of outpatient cardiovascular disease care: insights from the NCDR PINNACLE Registry. J Am Coll Cardiol 66(16):1803–1812

Woo BFY, Lee JXY, Tam WWS (2017) The impact of the advanced practice nursing role on quality of care, clinical outcomes, patient satisfaction, and cost in the emergency and critical care settings: a systematic review. Hum Resour Health 15(1):63. https://doi.org/10.1186/s12960-017-0237-9. PMID: 28893270; PMCID: PMC5594520

References

AANP (2015) https://storage.aanp.org/www/documents/advocacy/position-papers/ScopeOfPractice.pdf

Adamy EK, Zocche DAA, Almeida MA (2020) Contribution of the nursing process for the construction of the identity of nursing professionals. Rev Gaúcha Enferm 41(esp):e20190143. https://doi.org/10.1590/1983-1447.2020.20190143

Alshawush KA, Hallett N, Bradbury Jones C (2020) Impact of transition programmes for students and new graduate nurses on workplace bullying, violence, stress and resilience: a scoping review protocol. BMJ Open 10:e038893. https://doi.org/10.1136/bmjopen-2020-038893

Barnes H (2015) Exploring the factors that influence nurse practitioner role transition. J Nurse Pract 11(2):178–183. https://doi.org/10.1016/j.nurpra.2014.11.004

Berke NA (2018) Structured teaching can benefit all students. https://www.uft.org/news/teaching/teacher-teacher/structured-teaching-can-benefit-all-students? Accessed 22 Apr 2022

Blair K (Ed) (2019) advanced practice nursing roles. 6Th edition. Springer Publishing

Borrell-Carrió F, Suchman AL, Epstein RM (2004) The biopsychosocial model 25 years later: principles, practice, and scientific inquiry. Ann Fam Med 2(6):576–582. https://doi.org/10.1370/afm.245. PMID: 15576544; PMCID: PMC1466742

Bryant-Lukosius D, Martin-Misener R (2016) Advanced practice nursing: an essential component of country level human resources for health. ICN Policy Brief. https://www.who.int/workforcealliance/knowledge/resources/ICN_PolicyBrief6AdvancedPracticeNursing.pdf.   Accessed 20 Dec 2019

Darvill A, Stephens M, Leigh J (2018) Transition to nursing practice: from student to registered nurse. Sage Publishing, New York

Dlamini CP et al (2020) Developing and implementing the family nurse practitioner role in eswatini: implications for education, practice, and policy. Annual of Global Health 86(1):50,1–10. https://doi.org/10.5334/aogh.2813

Doucet TJ, Merlin MD (2014) Conceptualizations of health in nursing practice. Nurs Sci Q 27(2):118–125. https://doi.org/10.1177/0894318414522665. PMID: 24740946

Duchscher JB (2008) A process of becoming: the stages of new nursing graduate professional role transition. J Contin Educ Nurs 39(10):441–449

Dumphy D, DeSandre C, Thompson J (2019) Family nurse practitioner students' perceptions of readiness and transition into advanced practice. Nursing Forum 54:352–357. https://doi.org/10.111/nuf.12336

Faraz A (2016) Novice nurse practitioner workforce transition into primary care: a literature review. West J Nurs Res 38(11):1531–1545. https://doi.org/10.177/0193945916649587

Fitzgerald A (2020) Professional identity: a concept analysis. Nurs Forum 55:447–472. https://doi.org/10.1111/nuf.12450

Gysin S, Scottas B, Odermatt M, Essig S (2019) Advanced practice nurses' and general practitioners' first experiences with introducing the advanced practice nurse role to swiss primary care: a qualitative study. BMC Family Practice 20:163. https://doi.org/10.1186/s12875-019-1055-z

Haghighat S, Borhani F, Ranjbar H (2020) Is there a relationship between moral competencies and the formation of professional identity among nursing students? BMC Nurs 19:49. https://doi.org/10.1186/s12912-020-00440-y. PMID: 32536811; PMCID: PMC7288505

Halm MA (2021) Specialty certification: a path to improving outcomes. Am J Crit Care 30(2):156–160. https://doi.org/10.4037/ajcc2021569

Holt IGS (2008) Role transition in primary care settings. Quality in Primary Care 16:117–126

Hunter K, Cook C (2018) Role-modelling and the hidden curriculum: new graduate nurses' professional socialization. J Clin Nurs 27:3157–3170. https://doi.org/10.1111/jocn.14510

International Council of Nursing (2020) Guidelines on advanced practice nursing. Geneva. https://www.icn.ch/system/files/documents/2020-04/ICN_APN%20Report_EN_WEB.pdf. Accessed 17 Apr 2020

Kidner M (2019) APN role transition with leap leadership. Copyright of unpublished works. TXu 2-166-138. The United States Copyright Office

Maier CB, Barnes H, Aiken LH, Busse R (2016) Descriptive, cross-country analysis of the nurse practitioner workforce in six countries: size, growth, physician substitution potential. BMJ Open 6(9):e011901. https://doi.org/10.1136/bmjopen-2016-011901

Massaroli A, Martini JG, Moya JLM, Pereira MS, Tipple AFV, Maestri E (2019) Skills for generalist and specialist nurses working in the prevention and control of infections in Brazil. Rev Lat Am Enfermagem 27:e3134. https://doi.org/10.1590/1518-8345.2620.3134. PMID: 31038628; PMCID: PMC6528634

Moran GM, Nairn S (2018) How does role transition affect the experience of trainee advanced clinical practitioners: qualitative evidence synthesis. J Adv Nurs 74:251–262. https://doi.org/10.1111/jan.13446

Newhouse RP, Stanik-Hutt J, White KM, Johantgen M, Bass EB, Zangaro G, Wilson RF, Fountain L, Steinwachs DM, Heindel L, Weiner JP (2011) Advanced practice nurse outcomes 1990–2008: a systematic review. Nurs Econ 29(5):230–250; quiz 251. PMID: 22372080

Owens R (2019) Nurse Practitioner role transition and identity development in rural health care settings: a scoping review. Nursing Education Perspectives 40(3):157–161. https://doi.org/10.1097/01.NEP.0000000000000455

Pang SM, Wong TK, Wang CS, Zhang ZJ, Chan HY, Lam CW, Chan KL (2004) Towards a Chinese definition of nursing. J Adv Nurs 46(6):657–670. https://doi.org/10.1111/j.1365-2648.2004.03057.x. PMID: 15154907

Parse RR (2000) Paradigms: a reprise. Nurs Sci Q 13(4):275–276. https://doi.org/10.1177/08943180022107924. PMID: 11847744

Poghosyan L, Liu J, Norful AA (2017) Nurse practitioners as primary care providers with their own patient panels and organizational structures: a cross-sectional study. Int J Nurs Stud 74:1–7. https://doi.org/10.1016/j.ijnurstu.2017.05.004. Epub 2017 May 25. PMID: 28577459; PMCID: PMC6342506

Rasmussen P, Henderson A, Conroy T (2018) Factors influencing registered nurses' perceptions of their professional identity: an integrative literature review. J Contin Educ Nurs 49(5):225–232. https://doi.org/10.3928/00220124-20180417-08

Reynolds J, Mortimore G (2021) Transitioning to an ACP: a challenging journey with tribulations and rewards. Br J Nurs 30:3;166

Scott H (2002) RCN's definition of nursing: what makes nursing unique? Editorial. Br J Nurs 11(21):1356. https://doi.org/10.12968/bjon.2002.11.21.10922

Smith T, McNeil K, Mitchell R, Boyle B, Ries N (2019) A study of macro-, meso- and micro-barriers and enablers affecting extended scopes of practice: the case of rural nurse practitioners in Australia. BMC Nurs 18:14. https://doi.org/10.1186/s12912-019-0337

Tracy MF, O'Grady ET (eds.) (2019) Hamric and hanson's advanced practice nursing: an integrative approach, 6th ed. elsevier. ISBN:978-0-323-44775-1

Woo BFY, Lee JXY, Tam WWS (2017) The impact of the advanced practice nursing role on quality of care, clinical outcomes, patient satisfaction, and cost in the emergency and critical care settings: a systematic review. Hum Resour Health 15(1):63. https://doi.org/10.1186/s12960-017-0237-9. PMID: 28893270; PMCID: PMC5594520

Younas A (2020) Operationalist and inferentialist pragmatism: implications for nursing knowledge development and practice. Nurs Philos 21(4):e12323. https://doi.org/10.1111/nup.12323. Epub 2020 Aug 4. PMID: 32755025

Gaining Insight into Who You Will Become

2

2.1 Introduction

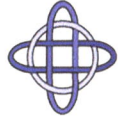

In this chapter you will begin the process of understanding the APN role and gaining an insight into who you will become as APN. This chapter will aid in the differentiation of the APN role from other nursing roles. The APN role has identified attributes and characteristics. Each will be discussed and applied to your structured APN role transition process. The common universal influences on the development of the APN include the sociopolitical environment, health needs of the country, the supply and demand of available healthcare workers, status of collaboration within nursing and other healthcare providers, and the development of the APN workforce within the country. The intent of this chapter is to expand your knowledge of the APN role and how the role works in your country.

Exemplar

Olivier is a specialist nurse in noncommunicable disease. He received his additional training in noncommunicable disease (NCD) management through a 3-month intensive training developed by the Ministry of Health and Partners in Health. After assuming the role as the specialist nurse running the NCD clinic he realized the benefit of becoming an APN along with his intense desire to be the nurse setting examples of the impact of nurses with an expanded scope of practice. Olivier enrolled in the university's graduate APN program where he is studying a new scope of practice and developing new systems in which APNs working in NCD can benefit the patients, community, and nursing.

M. Kidner, *Successful Advanced Practice Nurse Role Transition*, Advanced Practice in Nursing, https://doi.org/10.1007/978-3-030-53002-0_2

2.2 Definitions

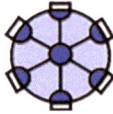

APN Characteristics Features or qualities that have been identified as common and universal in APNs worldwide and help make the role identifiable as APN are considered APN characteristics (Hutchinson et al. 2014; ICN 2020, p. 10).

APN responsibilities APN role obligations in which the APN accepts as a moral and legal accountability and part of the position as APN. APN responsibilities can be country specific (Carryer et al. 2007).

Assumptions of APNs In this context, it is assumed that all APN education programs have provided the students with the universal education required for APN practice and based within the context of nursing and nursing principle (ICN 2020, p. 9).

Nursing Paradigm Scientific paradigms provide fundamental thesis statement that determine research and shape behaviors, influences of social phenomena, and attitudes of professional groups (Deliktas et al. 2019). Nursing paradigms provide foundations to understand person, environment, health, and nursing developing a distinct discipline and unique knowledge base for both research and clinical practice (Deliktas et al. 2019; Donohue-Porter et al. 2017).

Professional (APN) efficacy Professional efficacy requires two components: (1) A set of evidence-based competencies required to structure the APN role and (2) the creation of personal confidence in the competencies and to uphold the profession's values and ethics creating a sense of belonging and strength in the embodiment of the role. In this book, professional efficacy is specific to the APN role (Gutierrez and Morais 2017; Hagighat et al. 2020).

Scope of practice The services that a qualified APN is permitted to undertake by regulations and deemed competent to perform. The scope of practice is made up of the activities APNs carry out within the professional role within your country. Your scope of practice is the limit of your knowledge, skills, and experience and is made up of the activities you carry out within your professional role (https://www.hcpc-uk.org/standards/meeting-our-standards/scope-of-practice/ accessed 22 April 2022).

Stakeholders Any individual or group that is impacted by the decisions or activities of an APN is a stakeholder for that APN (Concannon et al. 2014).

Values   Values are learned beliefs, attitudes that are learned and embedded in one's ethical systems that attempt to understand and model moral behaviors. Professional values are determinants of behavior and influence professional actions (Arries 2020; Coplu and Tekinsoy Kartın 2019; Schmidt and McArthur 2018).

2.3   A Day in Clinical Practice

Have you wondered what your clinical practice day will be like as an APN? It is natural to wonder. Exploring your past experiences can help to form your future ideal vision of an APN. The clinical practice for a generalist nurse is different than the clinical practice of the APN. Understanding the differences of the generalist nurse and APN will allow you to start the process of your role transition.

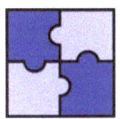

Describe a typical day at your current nursing practice location your roles, activities, required skills/knowledge, your current supervisory functions, and the common relationships required for work:

_____
_____
_____
_____
_____
_____
_____
_____
_____
_____
_____
_____
_____
_____

Now describe what you think a clinical practice day as an APN will be and how your clinical practice will be different from your current nursing role:

_____
_____
_____
_____

_____
_____
_____
_____
_____
_____
_____
_____
_____
_____
_____
_____

What are the differences and similarities in the day of clinical practice?

_____
_____
_____
_____
_____
_____
_____
_____

2.4   The APN Role

What is meant by the APN *role*? According to the Merriam dictionary (online), a "*role*" is a connected collection of specialized skills, knowledge, rights, behaviors, ethics, and standards held to be required to fulfill a social situation and socially expected behavior patterns usually determined by an individual's status in a particular society. The "role" of the APN is unique in different settings and countries because the inherent characteristic of "role" involves society. In some countries instead of a distinct nursing role, the APN may be considered a different "level" of nursing. No matter the word choice, the APN enhances the provision of healthcare services and can provide approaches for unmet needs by using the enhanced specialized knowledge, skills, standards, and behaviors developed within nursing and nursing ethics.

A structured process for role transition and the development of a professional identity encompasses the exploration of the APN role including the development of skills, knowledge, rights, behaviors, ethics, standards, and understanding of the APN role responsibilities. Your current experience as a generalist nurse will be enriched through graduate education, skills, and clinical experiences. Your APN education is an exciting opportunity to be creative and innovative in your workplace and your country. You may have opportunities to:

- Identify, imagine, and develop pathways for the APN role in your country
- Provide and expand access to care in your country
- Educate others on the APN role
- Build new relationships

If you are determined, you will have the capacity to develop the skills, knowledge, and behaviors to uphold the APN standards and responsibilities of the APN role.

2.4.1   Assumptions About APN

There are basic assumptions of APNs who have successfully completed their APN graduate education. The assumptions of the APN graduate education identified in the *Guidelines on Advanced Practice Nursing 2020* are based on APN education, clinical experiences, judgment, ethics, and decision-making ability, which state that all APNs:

- Have a foundation in nursing and are practitioners of nursing.
- Provide safe and competent patient care.
- Have APN jobs with increased level of capabilities and knowledge that are measurable beyond that of a generalist nurse.
- Have acquired the ability to explain and apply the theoretical, empirical, ethical, legal, care giving, and professional development required for APN practice.
- Have defined standards and competencies within the country and workplaces which are periodically reviewed and updated to maintain currency in practice.
- Are influenced and change by the global, demographical, social, political, economic, and technology milieu.
- Use research to impact an evidence-based clinical practice (ICN 2020).

2.4.2   Characteristics of APN

The activities in which APNs are involved have specific nursing characteristics and ethical principles that are common themes throughout the APN practice worldwide. These APN characteristics distinguish the APN role from the generalist, or specialized, nurse roles with respect to education, nature of practice, and regulatory mechanisms (ICN 2020). Understanding the characteristics that clearly define an advanced practice nurse increases the effective implementation of the role by clarifying the required skills, attributes, and knowledge required to implement the role completely (Hutchinson et al. 2014). These APN characteristics are inherent in the processes of developing/mentoring of others, improving systems of care, developing and delivering educational activities, being active in nursing research and scholarship, and implementing clinical leadership (Hutchinson et al. 2014).

When considering nursing activities of general, specialized, and advanced practice nurses one can see many activities/tasks/or skills are similar. All provide direct care to patients, all do physical exams, all can manage patients, and all can be excellent team members. Yet, the APN role has a significantly different knowledge base combined with an enhanced thinking ability and clinical leadership to consider multiple possible outcomes of the actions, plans, educations, and medication combined with the authority to change or augment plans to improve clinical outcomes and patient quality of life (Heinen et al. 2019). The APN role can be distinguished from other nursing and non-nursing healthcare role by the APN's use of:

- A holistic perspective based in nursing theory
- The formation of therapeutic partnerships with patients and all stakeholders
- Expert clinical performance and clinical leadership
- Reflective practice to aid decision-making and professional identity formation
- Evidence as a guide to practice while maintaining an understanding that all patients are unique people
- Diverse approaches to health and illness management (Tracy et al. 2019)

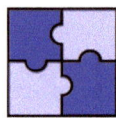

What characterizes APN?

What activities/characteristics make the APN role recognizable *as nursing*?

_____
_____
_____
_____
_____
_____
_____
_____

What activities/characteristics make the APN role *unique* in nursing?

_____
_____
_____
_____
_____
_____
_____

Following are some activities/characteristics of Advanced Practice Nursing:

- **Advanced APN knowledge and nursing expertise** from formal graduate education including:
  - Advanced pharmacology
  - Physiology and pathophysiology
  - Theories about human response to health
  - Building trust relationships with patients, families, and all stakeholders
  - Detailed history and physical assessments
  - Laboratory and diagnostic testing: ordering, interpreting, and making decisions based on the data
  - Differential diagnosis (medical and nursing)
  - Treatment and comprehensive healthcare plan development
  - Clinical leadership and leadership theories
  - Healthcare systems, teams and change theories/implementation
  - Clinical leadership at patient, team, and committee levels
  - Formal leadership role in teams, committees, organizations, and associations (local, national, and international)
  - Intra- and interprofessional teams, committees, members, and leaders
  - Research skills and statistics including translation of research into clinical practice
  - Use of evidence-based practice to create policy and procedures
  - Understanding and ability to impact policy and regulation to support and develop autonomous nursing practice at the top of the scope of practice (ICN 2020; Tracy et al. 2019; Heinen et al. 2019)

- **Advanced skills and competencies** are obtained through formal graduate education and clinical practicum requirements. These skills can vary from country to country depending on social determinants and process of APN role implementation. It is the combined ability to use critical thinking to the skill that makes the activity within the realm of the APN. Advanced skills and competencies *can* include:
  - Suturing of deep and multi-layered surgical and traumatic laceration closures
  - Electrocardiogram interpretations (rhythm strip and 12 leads) with subsequent plan of care/response to the 12 lead EKG
  - Ultrasounds and echocardiograms: ordering, conducting, and interpreting
  - Reproductive management and care
  - Emergency room skills
      Airway management and tracheal intubation
      Splinting, fracture stabilization
      Local anesthesia application
      Defibrillation/cardioversion
      Complex wound debridement and care
      Resuscitation and shock stabilization

  - Hemodynamic monitoring and stabilization
  - Removal of foreign bodies and abscess drainage and biopsy

– Performing consultations and authority for autonomous referrals
– Mental health evaluations and treatment plans
– Differentiates between exacerbation and reoccurrence of a chronic psychiatric disorder and signs and symptoms of a new mental health problem or a new medical or psychiatric disorder
– Diagnoses commonly occurring complications of mental health problems and psychiatric disorders, including physical health problems
– Evaluates the health impact of multiple life stressors and situational crises within the context of the family cycle
– Applies standardized taxonomy systems to the diagnosis of mental health problems and psychiatric disorders
– Differentiates psychiatric presentations of medical conditions from psychiatric disorders and arranges appropriate evaluation and follow-up
– Evaluates potential abuse, neglect, and risk of danger to self and others, such as suicide, homicide, and other self-injurious behaviors, and assists patients and families in securing the least restrictive environment for ensuring safety (Kleinpell et al. 2006; Kleinpell et al. 2014; Wiener 2016; https://www.allencollege.edu/filesimages/academics/PMHNP_Competencies.pdf accessed 22 April 2022)

• **Expert clinical judgment** obtained through formal graduate education and clinical practicum requirements is applied on an extended scope of practice in a variety of situations, including:
  – Complex healthcare plan design and management/evaluation
  – Systems management and change implementation/evaluation
  – Establishing evidence-based practice standards
  – Mentoring and monitoring clinician performance
  – Delegates and supervises tasks assigned to paraprofessional staff
  – Creates a culture of ethical standards within organizations and communities
  – Assumes a leadership role of an interprofessional healthcare team with a focus on the delivery of patient-centered care and the evaluation of quality and cost-effectiveness across the healthcare continuum
  – Team leadership, management, and capacity building
  – Plans and implements training and provides technical assistance and nursing consultation to health department staff, health providers, policy makers, and personnel in other community and governmental agencies and organizations
  – Research: conducting and implementing results
  – Complex patient case management (autonomously developed, implemented, and evaluated)
  – Urgent and emergent clinical care (Heinen et al. 2019; Hutchinson et al. 2014; ICN 2020, p. 10; Tracy et al. 2019)

• **Increased decision-making** skills obtained through formal graduate education and clinical practicum requirements utilizing nursing ethics, evidence-based practice, advanced nursing knowledge, and expert clinical judgment to provide high-quality healthcare to those within one's scope of practice. The ability to creatively and critically think on complex healthcare issues and processes from patient to systems is an essential hallmark of the APN. The impact and outcomes of this increased decision-making include:

– Simple to complex decisions impacting a single person to large systems, countries, and even internationally
– Enhanced critical and creative thinking with focus on outcome management and leadership
– Leading quality assurance projects for small teams to entire workplace
– Capacity building with all stakeholders through dynamic relationships building techniques
– Engaged in strategic planning for teams, committees, and workplace levels
– Audit and evaluation to improve practice in systems from simple processes to complex systems
– Understanding, implementation, and evaluation of evidence-based practices with translation to practical policy designs to the introduction of new clinical practices for teams, workplaces, or the country
– Enhanced knowledge and ability to design, conduct, and evaluate clinical research to enhance nursing and patient care outcomes (Heinen et al. 2019; Hutchinson et al. 2014)

• **Nature of APN Practice** is complex and can vary from country to country because APNs impact both direct and indirect services to patients and communities. APN practice is changing with APN research and the understanding of the high-quality care APNs provide in a variety of settings. Some APN activities that exemplify the dynamic nature of the APN role can include:

– Provides and supervises direct patient care at an advanced level
– Provides and supervises indirect patient care (such as case management, staff education, leadership, team building, community education, and needs assessments) at an advanced level through informal and formal leadership roles
– Provides comprehensive management of full episodes of care including the complex care of vulnerable and at-risk populations in chronic and acute illness/trauma using direct and indirect processes to ensure evidence-based nursing and outcomes management
– Ability to integrate evidence-based nursing research, education, leadership, and clinical management into comprehensive patient plans and healthcare systems
– Extended and broaden an in-depth range of autonomy through clinical expertise and trust relationships with stakeholders
– Ability to support and consult other healthcare providers emphasizing interprofessional and intraprofessional collaboration
– Ability to assess processes and systems to improve care through change and implementing evidence-based practices
– Can provide first point of contact for patients through an expanded scope of practice
– APNs as nurse anesthetists can provide anesthesia in operating theaters and pain management for simple and complex patients (ICN 2020, 2021; Tracy et al. 2019; Hutchinson et al. 2014)

- **Increased Authority** is granted through the country's formal and legal APN scope of practice. Activities involving an increased nursing authority include:
  - Authority to diagnose using medical diagnosis
  - Authority to prescribe and follow medications
  - Authority to determine need, order, and interpret diagnostic testing and therapeutic treatments
  - Authority to refer patients to other healthcare providers or services
  - Authority to admit and discharge patients from hospitals
  - Authority to use the APN title and work to full licensure (ICN 2020, p. 10)

- **Enhanced informal and formal leadership knowledge and skills** obtained throughout the graduate APN education and clinical practice. This increase in leadership and management is seen in many APN activities in direct and indirect patient care, including:
  - Guides, initiates, and provides leadership in policy-related activities to influence practice, health services, and public policy
  - Clearly articulates, exemplifies, and advocates the value of nursing to key stakeholders and policy makers
  - Provides leadership to the healthcare team to promote health, facilitate self-care management, optimize patient engagement, and prevent future decline including progression to higher levels of care and readmissions
  - Acts as a resource person, preceptor, mentor/coach, and role model demonstrating critical and reflective thinking
  - Uses positive communication skills/processes and emotional intelligence to lead quality improvement and patient safety initiatives in healthcare systems, build capacity, and increase trust with stakeholders
  - Assumes as a clinical expert, a leadership role in establishing and monitoring standards of practice to improve client care, including intra- and interdisciplinary peer supervision and review
  - Advocates for and participates in creating a workplace culture that supports safe patient care, collaborative practice, and professional growth
  - Supports knowledge application through evidence-based practice translation of research to clinical impact
  - Employs consultative, leadership, and emotional intelligence skills with intra-professional and interprofessional teams to create change in healthcare and complex healthcare delivery systems
  - Collaborates with healthcare professionals, including physicians, advanced practice nurses, nurse managers, and others, to plan, implement, and evaluate an improvement opportunity (Tracy et al. 2019; Heinen et al. 2019).

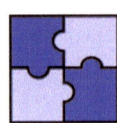

What aspects of the APN in your country characterizes the APN role as described above?

_____
_____
_____
_____
_____
_____
_____
_____

The list of characteristics, competencies, and features may be different based upon your culture, the educational system for nursing and the acceptance of the nursing profession in your country. Worldwide, nursing symbolizes these characteristics, values, and principles. You will continually develop your education and practice as an APN to enhance these core values. To work at your full scope of practice as an autonomous healthcare professional and provide benefit for your patients, it is important to understand these APN abilities and help your country obtain the legal authority for APNs to perform the skills that APNs have the education and experience to perform safely.

Ultimately what distinguishes the APN from other nursing roles is the expectation that every APN's clinical practice and leadership impacts will encompass all these competencies and seamlessly blend them into daily practice encounters with patients, colleagues, and stakeholders. This expectation makes APRN practice unique among that of other providers (Tracy et al. 2019).

Ethical principles are actions that support values and impact how a person, or group of people, will conduct themselves (Haddad and Geiger 2021). When ethical principles are developed and used for a profession, then these principles guide the professions' theory development, acceptable behaviors, research design and utilization, and professional growth (Haddad and Geiger 2021). Yet, to understand and embody nursing ethics as part of one's professional identity, one needs to understand how one gains such knowledge. Carpers' way of knowing is a process to understand and then use in a planned and structured process for clinical practice (Mantzorou and Mastrogiannis 2011; Rafii et al. 2021; Thorne 2020). For nursing, ethical principles address the nursing values of:

- Beneficence (do good for others)
- Nonmaleficence (do no harm)
- Dignity (treat everyone as worthy)
- Respect (Honor others' opinions, thoughts, feelings, wishes, rights, or traditions)
- Autonomy (ability to make correct decision by oneself)
- Social justice (equal economic, political, and social rights and opportunities)
- Professional practice (recognition of nursing as a distinct profession) (McDermott-Levy et al. 2018)

The focus of ethical principles encompasses the right and wrong during the complex decision-making process and accepting the ultimate consequences of those actions (Haddad and Geiger 2021). All levels of nursing (generalist, specialist, and advanced practice) use nursing ethical principles to base the care they provide to others. The consistent use of nursing ethical principles impacts the characteristics of the APN role. Therefore, it is important to take a quick review of nursing ethics. Currently, there are substantial pressures in healthcare that create challenges and stress in the workplace (such as staffing, increased acuity, a pandemic, and/or lack of supplies). Thus, the need for nurses to role model ethical care and ethical decisions is critical for patient outcomes and workplace morale (Hunter and Cook 2018).

An excellent resource to review when you are exploring Nursing ethics is the revised 2021 The ICN Code of Ethics for Nurses which can be found at: https://www.icn.ch/system/files/2021-10/ICN_Code-of-Ethics_EN_Web_0.pdf.

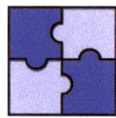

Ways of Knowing to Impact Ethics and Professional Identity
Personal knowing is the self-recognition and understanding of one's thoughts as it pertains to a topic or chosen profession. The building of this skills requires the use of nursing knowledge to be reflected upon in different viewpoints including one's own experiences, personal and professional values and ethics.

Carper's Way of Knowing (1970s)

1. **Empirical way of knowing** is formally expressed through facts, models, theories, and thematic descriptions. This is synonymous with science and provides a process to describe and explain social and natural phenomena. This includes nursing conceptual models and theories.
2. **Ethical way of knowing** focuses on the ethical components of nursing practice and tries to answer the question of what is right and what is responsible. To develop the moral component requires understanding and clarification of personal philosophical positions supported by one's moral judgment and proven through advocating for others. Ethical way of knowing allows you to explore the morals of decisions and evaluate motives, values, and character of self and others.
3. **Personal way of knowing** enables the nurse to identify his/her responses, strengths and weaknesses in a situation and to be aware of the individual biases affecting the quality of the nurse–patient relationship. Understanding self is a reflective and planned journey with significant changes during role transitions. Personal knowing allows a person to be authentic and develop a healthy professional identity.
4. **Aesthetic way of knowing** or the art of nursing is achieved through empathy, dynamic adaptation, and understanding of the components as a whole as well as the recognition of specific cases rather than holism. This type of knowing is

based on the emotional and intellectual experience of nursing/events. This experience is a combination of subjective emotions and objective knowledge which is enhanced through effective and therapeutic communications upheld as essential in nursing. The use of clinical judgment, critical thinking, and professional competency are aspects of the Aesthetic way of knowing.
Additions to the original four ways of knowing

5. **Sociopolitical way of knowing** (1995) was added as a process of understanding the sociopolitical context both within the patient–nurse dyad and nursing as a practice profession within unique cultures and societies.
6. **Emancipatory way of knowing** (2008) is a capacity for man to be aware of the society, culture, and political situation of society and to critically reflect on these issues. This critical awareness and reflection are needed for change towards social justice and the understanding of cultural/society inequities. The rational of exploring emancipatory knowing is to both understand injustice experiences and to be an active part of solutions to improve people's lives.

(Mantzorou and Mastrogiannis 2011; Rafii et al. 2021; Swift and Twycross 2020; Thorne 2020)

Ways of Knowing: Application of theory to Practice

Answer the question through each style of the ways of knowing. Write your answer in the boxes below.

Why is understanding your APN role transition important for patients?

Empirical way of knowing (the science of the APN role)	Esthetic way of knowing—the art of nursing (clinical judgment, critical thinking, professional competence)
Ethical way of knowing-morals associated with decisions (evaluation of motives, values, and character)	Personal way of knowing (of self and of the APN profession)
Sociopolitical way of knowing (your country and culture)	Emancipatory way of knowing

Actions to support the nursing ethics values include:

1. Promoting an environment in which the human rights, dignity, values, customs, and spiritual beliefs of the individual, family, and community are respected.
2. Advocating for equality and social justice in resource allocation, access to healthcare and other social and economic services.
3. Demonstrating professional values such as respectfulness, responsiveness, compassion, trustworthiness, and integrity.
4. Exemplifying values that show support of diversity of opinion, beliefs, culture, and perspectives.
5. Consistently maintaining standards of personal conduct, which reflect well on the profession and enhance its image and public confidence.
6. Striving to foster and maintain a practice culture promoting ethical behavior and open dialogue.
7. Demonstrating responsibility and accountability for nursing practice and for maintaining competence by continual lifelong learning.
8. Striving to promote safe working conditions for nurses worldwide.
9. Sustaining a collaborative and respectful trust relationships with coworkers in nursing and other fields.
10. Working in partnership with nurses, groups, and governmental and nongovernmental organizations from around the world.
11. Protecting privacy of both people and personal data.
12. Acting with justice for patients, communities, nursing, and all stakeholders.
13. Using autonomy in decision-making.
14. Providing precise and accurate caring (through nursing knowledge, skills, decision-making, and collaboration) with individual and professional competency.
15. Using honesty and integrity in all actions to provide positive support of others through mentorship and leadership activities (Haddad and Geiger 2021; Kidner 2019; McDermott-Levy et al. 2018; Shahriari et al. 2013).

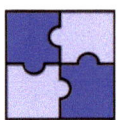

Activity In your opinion, what do you think is needed to be successful in those ethical activities? Consider the ethical principles that you believe all nurses and APNs should have. You can review the International Council of Nurses Code of Ethics at https://www.icn.ch/sites/default/files/inline-files/2012_ICN_Codeofethicsfornurses_%20eng.pdf.

_____
_____
_____
_____
_____
_____

_____

_____

_____

_____

Now consider yourself, what do you think you need to be able to uphold your values and nursing ethics in every action?

_____

_____

_____

_____

_____

_____

_____

_____

_____

As you gain additional insight on your personal resiliency and self-concept with this book, return to this question to ensure you have gained the skills and confidence through your professional identity development.

2.4.3   Scope of Practice of the APN

APN *scope of practice* identifies the range of services that have been determined that APNs are competent to perform and are permitted to provide to an identified population within their professional nursing credentialing and registration. Every country should have a specific APN scope of practice that is based on education, skills, and experience requirements that meet the needs of the country. Each specific APN role (CNS, NP, NA) requires a unique scope of practice based on the foundation of the appropriate advanced nursing education and professional standards for each specific APN role (ICN 2020).

It is important to understand the differences between the APN, specialist, and generalist scopes of practice (Gutierrez-Rodriguez et al. 2019). The APN completes a specific graduate-level education which includes autonomous advanced wholistic patient management (ICN 2020). It is this formal graduate education that is specifically designed for the APN role that separates the APN from the specialized and generalized nurse.

2.4.4   Developing an APN Scope of Practice

In each country, implementing the APN role needs to go through a process of scope of practice development. A well-established framework for APN role development is called PEPPA: a participatory, evidence-based, patient-focused process for APN role development (Bryant-Lukosius and DiCenso 2004). This model is unique as the patient-centered care is shaped by the relationships and roles of all stakeholders which are influenced by their respective values, beliefs, and experiences with APNs. Governmental and nongovernmental agencies have pivotal roles in defining how healthcare is provided to their citizens. The government's responsibility in healthcare includes:

1. Determining the types of healthcare providers designated to provide care to its citizens
2. Developing the scope of practice for healthcare providers
3. Providing resources for providers
4. Allowing healthcare professions access and engagement in health policy development (Morrison 2010).

Often countries develop the APN role in ad hoc processes by developing the education without stakeholders determining APN definitions, scope of practice, legal and regulatory requirements which ultimately impact professional identity and slow acceptance of the role in that country (Anderson et al. 2020; Heale and Buckley 2015). Both the scope of practice and the rules and regulations to implement the APN scope of practice will dramatically impact how the APN can practice and impact the health and wellness of others (Hudspeth and Kline 2019).

> ### *The developmental process of an APN scope of practice can include:*
>
> 1. Define patient population and current model of care.
> 2. Identify stakeholders and recruit participants from all stakeholder groups.
> 3. Nurses and stakeholders recognize an unmet health need, lack of healthcare providers, or process that can be fulfilled by an APN role.
> 4. Stakeholders evaluate resources, process, systems, and support to build a framework for that country.
> 5. Government officials are educated about APNs and potential to meet an unmet health need by providing high-quality care with recognized improved outcomes in other countries.
> 6. Determine the need and design of a new model of care (adding or expanding the APN role).
> 7. Identify priority problems, build solutions, and set goals through strategic planning.
> 8. Legislation is drafted and voted upon.
> 9. Government determines scope of practice (with education and guidance from healthcare experts—APNs must be present throughout the entire process).
> 10. Government then allows Ministers of Health and/or nursing boards to build the rules, regulations, and monitoring systems (Bryant-Lukosius & DiCenso 2004; Morrison, 2010).

The APN scope of practice document should be dynamic and change with the country's health needs, the changes in evidence-based practices, and new knowledge, skills, and technology that support the community's/country's health outcomes while maintaining care within the scope of practice (Hudspeth and Kline 2019; ICN Position Statement: Scope of Nursing Practice 2013; Morrison 2010).

The APN scope of practice is provided by the government and should support the expanded nursing role and provide or promote the pathway to autonomous APN practice (Morrison 2010). The written scope of practice should include the education requirements, and the full spectrum of roles, functions, responsibilities, activities and decision-making capacity that an individual within nursing is educated, competent, and authorized to perform. Most countries with successful APN practice have a clearly stated scope of practice.

A scope of practice should include:

- The specific APN role (NP, CNS, NA) for which the scope of practice was developed.
- The identity of the patient population in terms of complexity of healthcare that is to be the focus and comprehensiveness of services required.
- The professional accountability expected of the APN (obligation to perform at a competent level). This higher level of accountability promotes autonomy and is developed from the assumptions of the APN and the APN characteristics.
- The competencies required to fulfill the role. (Competencies are the application of the combination of knowledge, skills, building trust relationships, and decision-making.)
- The degree of accountability and authority that the healthcare provider assumes for practice outcomes (taking responsibility for one's actions). This degree of accountability and authority should clearly provide the agreed level of autonomy of the APN (Morrison 2010; Nieminen et al. 2011; Schober 2016, p. 67).

Scope of Practice Points for the APN Role of NP
The Nurse Practitioner (NP) is an APN who possesses advanced health assessment, diagnostic and clinical management skills that include pharmacology management based on additional graduate education (minimum standard master's degree) and clinical education that includes specified clinical practicum in order to provide a range of healthcare services. NP practice includes, but is not limited to, assessment; ordering, performing, supervising, and interpreting diagnostic and laboratory tests; making diagnoses; initiating and managing treatment including prescribing medication and non-pharmacologic treatments; coordinating care; counseling; and educating patients and their families and communities. The focus of NP practice is expert direct clinical care, managing healthcare needs of populations, individuals, and families, in outpatient/community or acute care settings with additional expertise in health promotion and disease prevention. As a licensed and credentialed clinician, the NP practices with a broader level of autonomy beyond that of a general, or specialized, nurse, advanced in-depth critical decision-making and works in collaboration with other healthcare professionals.

Key points of NP practice may include but is not limited to:

- Practicing autonomously and in coordination with healthcare professionals and other individuals.
- Providing a wide range of healthcare services including the diagnosis and management of acute, chronic, and complex health problems, health promotion, disease prevention, health education, and counseling to individuals, families, groups and communities.
- Serving as healthcare researchers, interdisciplinary consultants, and patient advocates.
- Base nursing decisions on nursing knowledge, evidence-based practice, skills, standards, and the needs of the patient.
- Integrating advanced knowledge of wellness, illness/disease, self-care, healthcare therapeutics in a holistic assessment of a person or a specific population while focusing on the nursing diagnosis of symptoms, functional problems, and risk behaviors that have etiologies requiring nursing interventions to prevent, maintain, or alleviate illness.
- Utilizing assessment data, research, and theoretical knowledge to design, implement, and evaluate nursing interventions that integrate delegated medical treatments as needed.
- Prescribing (ordering) and monitoring therapeutic interventions.
- Direct (autonomously) referral of patients to other services and professionals.
- Integrating of education, research, and leadership in conjunction with the emphasis on direct advanced clinical care.
- Provides clinical leadership within formal and informal leadership roles.

(American Association of Nurse Practitioners (AANP) n.d.-a, accessed 6/9/2021; ICN 2020; Kleinpell et al. 2014).

Scope of Practice Points for the APN Role of CNS

The CNS, identification of core competencies includes levels of direct and indirect nursing care. These levels of care include assisting other nurses and health professionals in establishing and meeting healthcare goals of individuals and a diverse population of patients.

Direct Care involves direct interactions with patients, families, and groups of patients to promote health or well-being and improve quality of life. Activities of direct care include:

- Integrates advanced knowledge of wellness, illness/disease, self-care, healthcare therapeutics in a holistic assessment of a person or a specific population while focusing on the nursing diagnosis of symptoms, functional problems, and risk behaviors that have etiologies requiring nursing interventions to prevent, maintain, or alleviate illness.

- Utilizes advanced assessment data, research, and theoretical knowledge to design, implement, and evaluate nursing interventions that integrate delegated medical treatments as needed.
- Prescribes or orders therapeutic interventions.

Indirect Care involves indirect provision of care through activities that influences patient care outcomes. A CNS providing indirect can include

- Serves as a consultant to other nurses and healthcare professionals in managing highly complex patient care problems and in achieving quality, cost-effective outcomes for populations across healthcare settings.
- Develops evidence-based guidelines or protocols for care and staff development activities.
- Provides leadership in appropriate use of research/evidence in practice innovations to improve healthcare services.
- Develops, plans and directs programs of care for individuals and populations and provides direction to nursing personnel and others in these programs of care.
- Evaluates patient outcomes and cost-effectiveness of care to identify needs for practice improvements.
- Serves as a leader of multidisciplinary groups in designing and implementing alternative solutions to patient care issues across the continuum of care. (ICN 2020)

2.4.5   APN as Nurse Anesthetist (NA)

There is a critical society unmet need to provide access to anesthesia and surgery for people who are needlessly suffering, disabled and dying because of lack of appropriately trained healthcare providers in anesthesia. For example, an estimated 808 women die each day due to complications of pregnancy and childbirth that needed surgical intervention (ICN 2021). The APN Nurse Anesthetist role developed to provide nurses the ability to provide high-quality, safe care increasing access to surgical procedures and complex pain therapies. NAs have the enhanced responsibilities and authorities of all APNs plus:

- Delivers anesthesia, pain management and related care with a high degree of autonomy in both independent and collaborative practices to patients of all ages and conditions
- Prepares, manages, and monitors all medications, materials, and equipment for all anesthesia procedures
- Has the authority to admit to hospitals
- Has the authority to practice to the full scope of nurse anesthesia practice (ICN 2021)

A Scope of Practice Points for the APN Role of NA

A Nurse Anesthetist (NA) is an APN (completing all APN focused graduate education) who has the knowledge, skills, and competencies to provide individualized care in anesthesia, pain management, and related anesthesia services to patients across the lifespan through all levels of acuity, including immediate, severe, or life-threatening illnesses or injury. NAs are involved in preoperative, intraoperative, and postoperative anesthesia care. They prepare and check anesthesia machines, monitors, drugs, materials, and equipment for all anesthesia procedures and airway management. NAs administer or participate in the administration of general and regional anesthesia to all ages and categories of patients and surgical procedures. They are responsible for a broad variety of anesthesia techniques, anesthetic agents, adjunctive and accessory drugs, as well as with pain management and safe sedation procedures. They conduct effective analysis and utilization of invasive and non-invasive monitoring data to autonomously adjust treatment plans as needed. NAs recognize and take appropriate action when complications/emergencies occur and immediately consult with appropriate others if patient safety requires it or if the incidence exceeds their scope of practice. They serve as provider and resource persons in cardiopulmonary resuscitation, respiratory care, and other acute care needs.

(https://www.aana.com/docs/default-source/practice-aana-com-web-documents-(all)/scope-of-nurse-anesthesia-practice.pdf?sfvrsn=250049b1_2 accessed 11 July 2020; International Federation of Nurse Anesthetists Code of Ethics, Standards of Practice, Monitoring, and Education 2016, accessed 11 July 2020; ICN 2021)

In some countries, CNS, NP, and NA roles may have prescriptive authority for medications and plans of care they also can refer patients to other healthcare providers. It is essential to know the laws of your country to understand the authority granted to you is based on your specific APN education, role, and scope of practice.

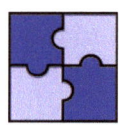

Thinking Points

Answer the following questions **as if APN role is in your country**:
Who do you provide healthcare to based upon your APN education?

_____

_____

What skills will/should you be able to autonomously provide to the population for whom you provide healthcare?

_____

_____

Why should you be granted the right to provide the above care?

_____

_____

Where can you provide your clinical services as APN? (hospitals, clinics, in public spaces, in homes)

_____

_____

What is the scope of APN practice in your country?

_____

_____

_____

_____

_____

_____

_____

_____

_____

_____

_____

_____

_____

_____

2.5   What Should Be the APN Professional Protected Title?

Your title is what clearly identifies you to patients and colleagues and optimally should be legally protected. It may seem simple, yet the process of a title has been complex. Internationally there has been a lack of consensus for one distinct and protected title for nurses working at an advanced level. This lack of defined title and definition of the role attached to the title adds confusion within and outside of nursing. Healthcare team relationships are vital to the APN role transition and title clarity promotes the development of these relationships (Faraz 2016). In many countries, the term "Advanced Practice" simply means nurses with nursing education beyond a bachelor's degree (Torrens et al. 2020). Currently with the 2020 ICN Guidelines on Advanced Practice Nursing there is a clarity to the term "APN." The international use of multiple titles can lead to lack of role clarity, inconsistent expectations, restrictive employer job descriptions, role conflict, role overload, and variable stakeholder acceptance (Healy and Buckley 2015).

In 2016, Schober found the following titles were used for those working in the advanced nursing practice role around the world:

- Nurse Practitioner (44%)
- APN (17%)

  – Advanced Practice Nurse
  – Advanced Practitioner of Nursing
  (Schober 2016; National Council of State Board of Nursing n.d.)
  Other titles used in different countries and jurisdictions within countries:
- Advanced Nurse Practitioner (ANP)
- Clinical Nurse Specialist (CNS)
- Nurse Specialist (NS)
- Professional Nurse (PN)
- Expert Nurse (EN)
- Certified Registered Nurse Practitioner (CRNP)
- Nurse Consultant (NC)
- Advanced Practice Registered Nurse (APRN)
- Advanced Registered Nurse Practitioner (ARPN)
- Advanced Practice Nurse Practitioner (APNP)
- Certified Nurse Practitioner (CNP)
  (Schober 2016; National Council of State Board of Nursing n.d.)

2.5.1   Title Confusion and Consensus

ICN released the new APN guidelines in 2020 and supports the title "APN." The APN title may not be internationally uniform until all the countries implementing the APN role adopt the recommended title. To be an advocate for the APN role, it is imperative to understand the APN definition and title within your country and at the international level (Torrens et al. 2020). If the title and associated role are not clearly defined, then role ambiguity in relationships with other clinical team members or barriers to practice can emerge (Kleinpell et al. 2014). Whereas a clear role, title, and scope of practice understanding will increase the ability to collaborate, develop trust relationships, and impact all stakeholders (Anderson et al. 2020; Torrens et al. 2020).

  Graduate education requirements, licensing and titling consensus has been difficult for many countries including the United States of America. It was not until 2008, the National Council of State Boards of Nursing APRN Advisory Committee and the APRN Consensus Work Group created the *APRN Consensus Model* in an effort to create consistence and clarity related to licensure, accreditation, certification, and education (*APRN* is used in the United States equivalent to APN used in other countries). The APRN roles identified are certified nurse midwife (CNM), certified registered nurse anesthetist (CRNA), clinical nurse specialist (CNS), and nurse practitioner (NP). The definition of an Advanced Practice Registered Nurse (APRN) outlined by the *Consensus Model* is detailed. The entire document can be found at: https://www.ncsbn.org/aprn-consensus.htm.

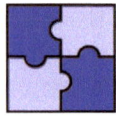

Thinking Points

Why is it important to have a clearly stated title?

_____
_____
_____
_____

What title(s) and associated scopes of practice are used in your country and is there a different education process for different scopes of practice?

_____
_____
_____
_____
_____
_____
_____
_____
_____
_____
_____

A consistent APN title in your country allows for a better understanding of both the role of the APNs and support the presence of APNs as healthcare providers. In addition, a consistent title helps the stakeholders and public understand what healthcare the APN provides and how APNs can impact the community. This is important because stakeholders and public do not always fully understand what services an APN can provide and under what circumstances when working at their full scope of practice.

2.6   APN Core Functions

APN implementation throughout the world is in a variety of stages with different titles, different scopes of practice, different regulations, and different levels of authority. This variation can lead to lack of role clarity, poor job description, inconsistent expectations, and variable stakeholder acceptance. This range of differences added to the complexities of role implementation has been revealed in the literature with common themes of APN functions (Carney 2016; Carryer et al. 2007; Heale et al. 2015). Although there are many functions of the APN, the following core functions are true for any APN in any setting (Carney 2016):

1. **Creating and promoting a dynamic clinical practice to improve patient outcomes**—Autonomous or nurse-led extended clinical practice is the primary influence in a creative and dynamic workplace environment. The APN practice

is built upon previous nursing knowledge encompassing an extensive, evidence-based and systematic clinical knowledge and skill set with the ability to apply the knowledge and skills with concerns to both clinical and social contexts.
This dynamic practice includes:

(a) Patient assessments
(b) Direct patient care
(c) Initiative therapy
(d) Ordering and interpreting investigative procedures
(e) Translating evidence-based research into clinical practice
(f) The use of technology
(g) Clinical leadership
(h) System analysis and clinical system changes
(i) Policy development
(j) Interprofessional team collaboration

(Carney 2016; Hutchinson et al. 2014).

2. **Developing and promoting APN professional efficacy**—The increased knowledge and skills are delivered through nursing frameworks (such as biopsychosocial, humanbecoming paradigm, totality, and simultaneity models). A cornerstone of APN care is linked to the nursing framework where APNs seek meaningful encounters with every patient incorporating the maximization of individual's well-being through understanding the person's social context and personal desires to develop mutually agreed plans. Professional efficacy includes understanding self through multiple processes of knowing (Carper's ways of knowing), reflective practice to understand self as APN, and building capacity through the development of stakeholder's trust through the daily implementation of decisions based on nursing ethic principles combined with effective communication competencies. In addition, APN professional efficacy includes all activities pertaining to career development and societal acceptance/support of the APN role locally, nationally, and internationally (Anderson et al. 2020; Carney 2016; Haghighat et al. 2020).

3. **Developing and sustaining APN clinical leadership**—APN clinical leadership is evident when APNs autonomously develop treatment processes in complex healthcare situations, exert positive influence, develop and implement change strategies, consult, mentor, educate, collaborate, and establish trust relationships with other health professionals and formal leaders (Blanck-Köster et al. 2020). The core function of clinical leadership develops from a strong base of graduate education and clinical experience. Combined with an awareness of the importance of nursing within the healthcare systems of the country, this leadership includes both formal and informal roles. APNs combine their strong patient and staff advocacy with profession-focused support at multiple system levels within the country's healthcare structure. Clinical leadership is enhanced through the increased knowledge of advanced assessments, pathophysiology, data interpretation, diagnostic skills, and pharmacology knowledge (Lamb et al. 2018).

2.7   Influences on the Development of the APN Role

Whether your country established the APN role years ago, or is newly developing the APN role, it takes advocates and stakeholders who can anticipate the potential impact of APNs to society to successfully implement the APN role. Advocacy and time are required to pass legislation, regulation, and professional standards which can build the scope of practice in professional and legal terms. It is essential for APNs to understand that governmental legislation permits the APN role to your country followed by the subsequent development of regulations to guide the implementation of that role. Research on common forces that impact the stakeholder's vision of potential APN impact and role development include:

1. **The sociopolitical environment**

   (a) The combination of the country's current ideologies, regulations, policies, conditions, laws, practices, and traditions combined with social issues such as wealth, religion, buying habits, education level, family size and structure, and population density plus the past history, wars, and changes within the nursing profession is the sociopolitical environment (Ketefian et al. 2001; Raiesifar et al. 2016).

   (b) The sociopolitical environment of the country (how are the laws made, who has power, how is society treated by the government) (Schober 2016).

   (c) The public opinion of nursing impacts the success of the APN role implementation. Public perceptions are linked to the public's understanding of what nurses, including APNs, do in clinical practice. Many people do not recognize the complexity and scope of practice of nursing and the increased responsibility, accountability, and authority of the APN (Girvin et al. 2016). In many countries, the public perception of the nursing role is directly linked to the treatment of women (Sheer and Wong 2008).

2. **Health needs in society**

   (a) The community or country infrastructure for clean water, fresh food sources, proper sewer, proper garbage collection and disposal, housing, endemic diseases, pandemics, genetic disease prevalence, and prevalence of chronic noncommunicable diseases (diabetes, hypertension, heart disease, thyroid disease, chronic kidney disease, and liver disease) impacts the need for the APN role (Baguma 2017; Bouabid and Louis 2015; Ketefian et al. 2001; Li 2017; Mara et al. 2010).

   (b) The culture of current healthcare delivery (who provides healthcare where; what education is required; what is the level of acceptance, accountability, and responsibility) impacts the acceptance of the role (Schober 2016).

   (c) The response to the need to increase access to care with a focus on addressing disparities with the consideration of social, cultural, educational, and health circumstances of the population (Bryant-Lukosius and Martin-Misener 2016).

3. **Health workforce supply and demand**

   (a) This includes the current number of physicians caring for the population, staffing of hospital and clinics, the society understanding and trust of nursing, and the need for more healthcare providers (physicians/APNs) in hospitals, clinics, and public health agencies in the country (Ketefian et al. 2001; Morrison 2010; Xue et al. 2016).

   (b) The awareness of current and potential APN impact to the healthcare delivery system by key stakeholders and decision makers (understanding of the role of APNs as healthcare providers, and roles the APN has, the potential impact to patients, families, and society) increases the role awareness (Xue et al. 2016).

4. **Governmental policy and support**

   (a) The level of governmental support to develop the APN role through legislative activities impacts the speed in which the role can be developed within a country.

   (b) Provides the process to develop the APN scope of practice; continual support to monitor progress to the APN role to full-practice authority (the ability to work autonomously without physician control/supervision) (Heale and Rieck 2015; Ketefian et al. 2001).

   (c) Changes in legislation, policy, and healthcare reform (how do other healthcare providers react; how do legislators react; and how do nurses advocate for change) are related to the support legislators and governmental officials may offer (Schober 2016).

5. **Intraprofessional (nursing) and interprofessional collaboration for maximum effectiveness of the advanced role**

   (a) The organizations collaborating with nurses, physicians, and other healthcare providers to develop processes for integrated care (Carney 2016; Heale and Rieck 2015; Heinen et al. 2019; Ketefian et al. 2001).

   (b) This collaboration should maximize the potential impact of APN clinical expertise and leadership on illness, wellness, and disease prevention for patients, communities, country and international levels.

   (c) International organization support for interprofessional collaboration in healthcare (Schober 2016). Such as
   - World Health Organization
   - International Council of Nurses
   - World health Professional Alliance
   - Pan American Health Organization
   - Sigma Theta Tau

   (d) Role ambiguity has allowed workplace senior executives to shape the APN role which often results in underutilization and inconsistent practices (Woo et al. 2019). In countries where the APN role was introduced in an ad hoc fashion with a lack of clear role definition and scope of practice, there are increased challenges related to role ambiguity through all stakeholders (Bryant-Lukosius and Martin-Misener 2016).

6. **The development of a highly skilled and educated nursing workforce to provide the needed access to care** (Bryant-Lukosius and Martin-Misener 2016; Carryer et al. 2007; Morrison 2010; Xue et al. 2016). The ICN 2020 guidelines has established the APN education as masters or doctoral.

   (a) A global effort to increase access to care through nursing using nursing theories and a biopsychosocial model to create patient-centered care that includes both technical and advanced education in a wellness paradigm.
   (b) Allows for advanced career development in nursing.
   (c) Curriculum development considering role implementation and society needs.
   (d) APNs are significant influencers to the development of the APN role. Important contributions of the daily activities of APNs include (Woo et al. 2019):

       • Providing detailed education and counseling to staff and stakeholders
       • Providing practical and realistic patient education
       • Providing direct comprehensive patient-centered care
       • Building and maintaining therapeutic relationships and strong rapport with all stakeholders
       • Bridging the healthcare gaps with designing creative processes
       • Conducting nursing rounds
       • Revising policy and procedures with evidence-based information
       • Improving quality of care
       • Increasing access to care
       • Improving public perception of nursing

An excellent resource for gaining insight on the global development of the APN role:
   Global strategy on human resources for health: Workforce 2030 https://www.who.int/publications/i/item/9789241511131 7 July 2020

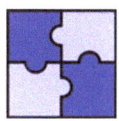

Consider and discuss each influence impacting the APN profession in relationship to your workplace, your professional identity, and your successful transition into the APN role.

_____
_____
_____
_____

_____
_____
_____
_____
_____
_____
_____
_____
_____
_____
_____
_____
_____
_____
_____

You may be a pioneer forging a brand-new path for nursing in your country. Your education experiences and future need to be informed by a precise understanding of potential challenges and ways for you to successfully overcome them. Understanding the scope of practice developmental process, knowing your governmental legislation and your country's rules and regulations concerning your APN role are most helpful in becoming a highly successful APN.

2.8   Stakeholders

A *stakeholder* is any person, or group of people, who have a valid interest in the profession/workplace and who will be impacted by you or will impact you or the country's APN role. Positive stakeholder engagement helps to align the needs of the society, healthcare providers, patients, policy makers, payors (insurance/government), and workplaces (Concannon et al. 2014). The importance of understanding stakeholders includes:

1. Creating and understanding the value of the APN role and your potential positive impact on others by seeking insight and information from stakeholders thereby sharing knowledge and resources together to promote APN value (Freeman et al. 2018).
2. Enhancing innovations in the APN integration into a variety of healthcare systems through the identification of the most relevant internal and external stakeholders to gather information and gain acceptance from those stakeholders (Freeman et al. 2018).

3. Developing interconnectivity with diverse stakeholders to increase the understanding and implementation of the APN role with greater society acceptance due to the diversity of stakeholders. This interconnectivity is dependent upon authenticity, and trust relationships (Freeman et al. 2018).
4. Improving relevance of research questions/quality improvement project with wide perspectives, enhanced transparencies, appropriate framing, and accelerated adoption of evidence into practice (Concannon et al. 2014).

It is relevant to role transition to ask yourself, "Who are the stakeholders for nursing and the APN role in my workplace and my country?"

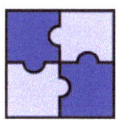

Make a list of all the people, or groups of people who are impacted by APNs, or who impact the success/failure of the APN role in your country. Next to each person's name/group identify why they are stakeholders. A short list of potential stakeholders is provided at the end of this chapter. You will be using this list later in the book for strategic planning (Chap. 6) and role transition.

_____
_____
_____
_____
_____
_____
_____
_____
_____
_____
_____
_____
_____
_____
_____
_____

"I didn't think that we were involved in great change...
but then change became the name of the game."
-Loretta Ford, 2011

2.9   APNs Impacting Health Worldwide

Advanced practice nursing (including the NP, CNS, and CRNAs) has grown due to the continued unmet patient needs, changing workforce needs, and increasing national and sociopolitical support of the role. The NP role expanded across the globe with the United States (1965), Canada (1970s), and Jamaica (1970s) as the first countries to implement the NP as primary healthcare providers to vulnerable, underserved, and/or rural populations (ICN 2020). In the 1980s, Botswana instituted the Family Nurse Practitioner role (ICN 2020) in Africa with the Kingdom of Eswatini implementing the Family Nurse Practitioner role in 2017 (Dlamini et al. 2020). Currently over 70 countries have implemented or are in the process of fully developing the APN role in their country (ICN 2020).

Countries are in different stages, with different governmental legislation creating different scopes of practice and using different titles. Yet the common attributes of a graduate education, a dynamic practice, professional efficacy, and clinical leadership remain common threads. Many regulatory systems are balancing public safety and licensing (or registration) of the APN with professional standards and supportive regulations/legislation (Carney 2016). The multiple titles, scope of practice, rules and regulations, and lack of knowledge of the APN role by decision makers and stakeholders can impact health outcomes (Carney 2016). Therefore, APN students can influence the future of the role through understanding and sharing the role, scope of practice, increased accountability, responsibility and authority, and the acceptable APN skills to all the stakeholders who impact role development in their country.

This section will be driven by the student (you) to allow for the most current data in your country to be incorporated. Countries that have implemented the APN role did so to address unique perspectives and factors impacting APN role development. These perspectives include the:

- Health needs of the society
- Culture of current healthcare delivery
- Healthcare workforce
- Sociopolitical environment of the country (wars, recessions, famines, disease outbreaks)
- Public opinion of nursing
- Awareness of APN impact by key stakeholders and decision makers
- Legislation, policy, and healthcare reform (government role and nursing regulatory boards)
- International organization support (i.e., International Council of Nurses) (Ketefian et al. 2001; Morrison 2010; Schober 2016)

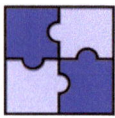

Activity   As an individual, or in small groups, complete the APN review for *your country*:

Develop a short presentation of 5–7 min including:
(a) The country description (location, population, any significant attributes and/or industry, basic economy, and primary health issues)
(b) The year the APN role started
   • What do you think was the motivator or the role development?
(c) Progress of the implementation of the APN role
(d) Comment on at least two of the five areas of influence:
   • The sociopolitical environment
   • Health needs in society
   • Health workforce supply and demand
   • Governmental policy and support
   • Intraprofessional (nursing) and interprofessional collaboration of effectiveness of the advanced role
(e) Describe how, with your review of the country, the APN role has benefited (any outcomes):
   • Society
   • Nursing

Notes on your country

_____
_____
_____
_____
_____
_____
_____
_____
_____
_____
_____
_____
_____
_____
_____
_____
_____
_____
_____
_____
_____

2.10   Local Culture and Impact

Your local and national culture concerning health, well-being, and illness plus the perception of nursing will directly impact the success of APNs in your area (Sheer and Wong 2008). Again, each area is highly specific, therefore this topic will be presented by students.

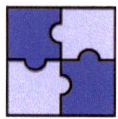

Group discussion points: Identify the differences and similarities between your country and the ICN Guidelines on Advanced Practice Nursing 2020 found at https://www.icn.ch/system/files/documents/2020-04/ICN_APN%20Report_EN_WEB.pdf

_____
_____
_____
_____
_____
_____
_____
_____
_____
_____
_____
_____
_____
_____
_____
_____
_____
_____
_____

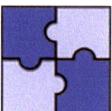

Learning from other countries. More than 70 countries have developed the APN role. This assignment can be done as an individual, or in groups of 2–4 people. https://international.aanp.org/Practice/Profiles and https://international.aanp.org/Research/SG are excellent websites that can provide you with information on several countries (or conduct an internet search).

Chose a country, other than your country. Each student/group must have a different country.

1. Develop a short presentation of 5–7 min including:

    (a) The country description (location, population, any significant attributes and/or industry, basic economy, and primary health issues)
    (b) The year the role started
        • What do you think was the driver (the unmet need) for APN role development?
    (c) Progress of the implementation of the APN role
    (d) Cultural similarities and differences with your country
    (e) If possible, comment on at least two of the five areas of influence.
        • The sociopolitical environment
        • Health needs in society
        • Health workforce supply and demand
        • Governmental policy and support
        • Intraprofessional (nursing) and interprofessional collaboration of effectiveness of the advanced role
    (f) Describe how, with your review of the country, the APN role has benefited (any outcomes):
        • Society
        • Nursing

_____
_____
_____
_____
_____
_____
_____
_____
_____
_____
_____
_____
_____
_____
_____

2.11   Summary

This chapter provides you with insights into who you are going to become as an APN by exploring the differences of generalist/specialist nursing and the APN role. This exploration starts by a comparison of a typical day of your practice as a generalist or specialist nurse and a day you envision as an APN. Although you will identify as a nurse, there are significant differences in the work of a nurse and that of an APN with increased responsibility, accountability, and authority based upon the advanced education and APN role. The 2020 ICN APN Guidelines defines three APN roles: the clinical nurse specialist (CNS), nurse practitioner (NP), and nurse anesthetist (NA). Each is discussed and a specific scope of practice is provided. This chapter provides a discussion on the assumptions, characteristics, and core functions of an APN. There are common influences that impact the development of the APN role worldwide. The six main influences on the APN role development influencers are:

- The sociopolitical environment
- Health needs of the society
- Health workforce supply and demands
- Governmental policy and support
- Intraprofessional (nursing) and interprofessional collaboration for maximum effectiveness of the APN role
- Development of highly skilled and educated APN workforce

Those influences involve stakeholders. Positive stakeholder engagement helps to align the needs of the society, healthcare providers, patients, policy makers, payors (insurance/government), and workplaces to support and advocate for the APN role. Lastly, this chapter expands to a global viewpoint of attributes and impact to health worldwide. The understanding of your country's APN role and impact is kept relevant through student discussions followed by peer presentations on other countries implement the APN role.

Appendix: Stakeholders

A "stakeholder" is any person, or group of people, who can impact the APN role, or who the APN will impact. It is important to recognize all stakeholders can impact in either positive or negative ways.

A list of possible APN stakeholders includes:

- Academic institutions and the upper leadership of directors and deans
- Instructors of the didactic courses
- Clinical instructors/preceptors
- Minister of Health
- A national board of nursing

- The country's political leader
- The country's governing body
- Hospital administrative staff
- Physicians
- Nurses
- Pharmacists
- Adjunct workplace staff: physical therapy, respiratory therapy, occupational therapy, dietary, housekeeping, billing
- Patients and their families
- Your community
- Public health agency and staff
- Nursing organizations: local, national, and international organizations

References

American Association of Nurse Practitioners (AANP) (n.d.-a) Scope of practice. https://www. aanp.org/advocacy/advocacy-resource/position-statements/scope-of-practice-for-nurse-practitioners. Accessed 27 Jan 2019

American Association of Nurse Practitioners (AANP) (n.d.-b) Quality of the NP. https://www. aanp.org/advocacy/advocacy-resource/position-statements/quality-of-nurse-practitioner-practice. Accessed 9 Apr 2020

American Nurses Association (ANA) (n.d.). https://www.nursingworld.org/practice-policy/scope-of-practice/. Accessed 27 Jan 2019

Anderson H, Birks Y, Adamson J (2020) Exploring the relationship between nursing identity and advanced nursing practice: an ethnographic study. J Clin Nurs 29:1195–1208. https://doi.org/10.1111/jocn.15155

Arries EJ (2020) Professional values and ethical ideology: perceptions of nursing students. Nurs Ethics 27(3):726–740. https://doi.org/10.1177/0969733019889396

Baguma D (2017) Public health safety and environment in inadequate hospital and healthcare settings: a review. Public Health 144:23–31. https://doi.org/10.1016/j.puhe.2016.11.014. Epub 2016 Dec 26. PMID: 28274380

Blanck-Köster K, Roes M, Gaidys U (2020) Clinical-Leadership-Kompetenzen auf der Grundlage einer erweiterten und vertieften Pflegepraxis (Advanced Nursing Practice): Ein Scoping-Review [Clinical leadership competencies in advanced nursing practice: Scoping review]. Med Klin Intensivmed Notfmed. Sep;115(6):466–476. German. https://doi.org/10.1007/s00063-020-00716-w. Epub 2020 Sep 1. PMID: 32870328

Bouabid A, Louis GE (2015) Capacity factor analysis for evaluating water and sanitation infrastructure choices for developing communities. J Environ Manag 161:335–343. https://doi.org/10.1016/j.jenvman.2015.07.012. Epub 2015 Jul 20. PMID: 26203872

Bryant-Lukosius D, DiCenso A (2004) A framework for the introduction and evaluation of advanced practice nursing roles. Nursing and health care management and policy. Blackwell Publishing LTD. In Advanced Practice Nursing Role: part II 530–540

Bryant-Lukosius D, Martin-Misener R (2016) Advanced practice nursing: an essential component of country level human resources for health. ICN Policy Brief. https://www.who.int/workforcealliance/knowledge/resources/ICN_PolicyBrief6AdvancedPracticeNursing.pdf. Accessed 20 Dec 2019

Carney M (2016) Regulation of advanced nurse practice: its existence and regulatory dimensions from an international perspective. J Nurs Manag 24:105–114

Carryer J, Gardner G, Dunn S, Gardner A (2007) The core role of the nurse practitioner: practice, professionalism and clinical leadership. J Clin Nurs 16:118–1825. https://doi.org/10.1111/j.1365-2702.2007.01823.x

Concannon TW, Fuster M, Saunders T, Patel K, Wong JB, Leslie LK, Lau J (2014) A systematic review of stakeholder engagement in comparative effectiveness and patient-centered outcomes research. J Gen Intern Med 29(12):1692–1701. https://doi.org/10.1007/s11606-014-2878-x

Coplu M, Tekinsoy Kartın P (2019) Professional self-concept and professional values of senior students of the nursing department. Nurs Ethics 26(5):1387–1397. https://doi.org/10.1177/0969733018761171

Deliktas A, Korukcu O, Aydin R, Kabukcuoglu K (2019) A nursing students' perceptions of nursing metaparadigms: a phenomenological study. J Nurs Res 27;5:1–9

Dlamini CP et al (2020) Developing and implementing the family nurse practitioner role in Eswatini: implications for education, practice, and policy. Annu Global Health 86(1):50. https://doi.org/10.5334/aogh.2813. 1–10

Donohue-Porter P, Forbes M, White J, and Baumann S. Transforming (2017) Nursing Education and the Formation of Students: Using the Humanbecoming Paradigm. Nurs Sci Q 30(2):134–142. https://doi.org/10.1177/0894318417693287

Faraz A (2016) Novice Nurse Practitioner Workforce transition into primary care: a literature review. West J Nurs Res 38(11):1531–1545. https://doi.org/10.1177/0193945916649587

Freeman E, Harrison J, Zyglidopoulos S (2018) Stakeholder theory. Cambridge University Press, Cambridge. https://doi.org/10.1017/9781108539500

Girvin J, Jackson D, Hutchinson M (2016) Contemporary public perception of nursing: a systematic review and narrative synthesis of the international research evidence. J Nurs Manag 24:994–1006. https://doi.org/10.1111/jonm.12413

Gutierrez MGR, Morais SCRV (2017) Systematization of nursing care in the formation of professional identity. Rev Bras Enferm 70(2):436–442. https://doi.org/10.1590/0034-7167-2016-0515

Gutierrez-Rodriguez L, Garcia Mayor S, Cuesta Lozano D, Burgos-Fuentes E, Rodreguez-Gomez S, Sastre-Fullana P et al (2019) Competencias en enfermeras Especialistas y en Enfermeras de Practicia Avanzada. Enferm Clin 29:328–335. https://doi.org/10.1016/j.enfcli.2019.01.001

Haddad LM, Geiger RA (2021) Nursing ethical considerations. [Updated 2020 Sep 1]. In: StatPearls [Internet]. StatPearls Publishing, Treasure Island. https://www.ncbi.nlm.nih.gov/books/NBK526054/

Haghighat S, Borhani F, Ranjbar H (2020) Is there a relationship between moral competencies and the formation of professional identity among nursing students? BMC Nurs 19:49. https://doi.org/10.1186/s12912-020-00440-y

Heale R, Rieck BC (2015) An international perspective of advanced practice nursing regulation. Int Nurs Rev 62(3):421–429. https://doi.org/10.1111/inr.12193

Heinen M, van Oostveen C, Peters J, Vermeulen H, Huis A (2019) An integrative review of leadership competencies and attributes in advanced nursing practice. J Adv Nurs 75(11):2378–2392 https://doi.org/10.1111/jan.14092. Epub 2019 Jul 21. PMID: 31162695; PMCID: PMC6899698

Hudspeth RS, Klein TA (2019) Understanding nurse practitioner scope of practice: regulatory, practice, and employment perspectives now and for the future. J Am Assoc Nurse Pract 31(8):468–473. https://doi.org/10.1097/JXX.0000000000000268. PMID: 31348141

Hunter K, Cook C (2018) Role-modelling and the hidden curriculum: new graduate nurses' professional socialization. J Clin Nurs 27:3157–3170. https://doi.org/10.1111/jocn.14510

Hutchinson M, East L, Stasa H, Jackson D (2014) Deriving consensus on the characteristics of advanced practice nursing: meta-summary of more than 2 decades of research. Nurs Res 63(2):116–128. https://doi.org/10.1097/NNR.0000000000000021. PMID: 24589642

ICN Position Statement: Scope of Nursing Practice (2013) https://www.icn.ch/sites/default/files/inline-files/B07_Scope_Nsg_Practice.pdf retrieved April 15, 2019

International Council of Nursing. Guidelines on Advanced Practice Nursing 2020 (2020) Geneva. https://wwwicnch/system/files/documents/2020-04/ICN_APN%20Report_EN_WEB.pdf. Accessed 17 Apr 2020

International Council of Nurses Guidelines on Advanced Practice Nursing Nurse Anesthetists 2021 (2021) Geneva. https://wwwicnch/system/files/2021-07/ICN_Nurse-Anaesthetist-Report_EN_WEBpdf. Accessed 18 Apr 2022

International Federation of Nurse Anesthetists Code of Ethics, Standards of Practice, Monitoring, and Education (2016). https://ifna.site/etusivu/practice/ifna-standards/. Accessed 11 Jul 2020

Ketefian S, Redman R, Hanucharurmkul S, Materson A, Neves E (2001) The development of advanced practice roles: implications in the international nursing community. Int Nurs Rev 48:152–163

Kidner M (2019) APN role transition with LEAP leadership. Copyright of unpublished works. TXu 2-166-138. The United States Copyright Office

Kleinpell R, Hravnak M, Werner K, Guzman A (2006) Skills taught in acute care NP programs: a national survey. Nurse Pract 31(2):7–13

Kleinpell R, Scanlon A, Hibbert D, Ganz F, East L, Fraser D, Wong F, Beauchesne M (2014) Addressing issues impacting advanced nursing practice worldwide. Online J Issues Nurs 19(2):5. https://doi.org/10.3912/OJIN.Vol19No02Man05

Lamb A, Martin-Miesner R, Bryant-Lukosius D, Latimer M (2018) Describing the leadership capabilities of advanced practice nurses using a qualitative descriptive study. Nurs Open 5:400–413. https://doi.org/10.1002/nop2.150

Li AM (2017) Ecological determinants of health: food and environment on human health. Environ Sci Pollut Res Int 24(10):9002–9015. https://doi.org/10.1007/s11356-015-5707-9. Epub 2015 Nov 10. PMID: 26552789; PMCID: PMC7089083

Mantzorou M, Mastrogiannis D (2011) The value and significance of knowing the patient for professional practice, according to the Carper's patterns of knowing. Health Sci J 5(4):251–261. E-ISSN: 1791-809X

Mara D, Lane J, Scott B, Trouba D (2010) Sanitation and health. PLoS Med 7(11):e1000363. https://doi.org/10.1371/journal.pmed.1000363

McDermott-Levy R, Leffers J, Mayaka J (2018) Ethical principles and guidelines of global health nursing practice. Nurs Outlook 66(5):473–481. https://doi.org/10.1016/j.outlook.2018.06.013

Morrison A (2010) Scope of nursing practice and decision-making framework TOOLKIT. ICN Regulation Series. https://www.icn.ch/sites/default/files/inline-files/2010_ICN%20Scope%20of%20Nursing%20and%20Decision%20making%20Toolkit_eng.pdf

Nieminen AL, Mannevaara B, Fagerström L (2011) Advanced practice nurses' scope of practice: a qualitative study of advanced clinical competencies. Scand J Caring Sci 25(4):661–670. https://doi.org/10.1111/j.1471-6712.2011.00876.x

Rafii F, Nasrabadi AN, Tehrani FJ (2021) How nurses apply patterns of knowing in clinical practice: a grounded theory study. Ethiop J Health Sci 31(1):139–146. https://doi.org/10.4314/ejhs.v31i1.16. PMID: 34158761; PMCID: PMC8188100

Raiesifar A, Firouzkouhi M, Fooladi M, Parvizy S (2016) Sociopolitical development of the nursing profession in Iran: a historical review. J Med Ethics Hist Med 9:13. PMID: 28050243; PMCID: PMC5203682

Schmidt BJ, McArthur EC (2018) Professional nursing values: a concept analysis. Nurs Forum 53:69–75. https://doi.org/10.1111/nuf.12211

Schober M (2016) Introduction to advanced nursing practice: an international focus, vol 1. Springer International, Basel, pp 63–64, 67

Shahriari M, Mohammadi E, Abbaszadeh A, Bahrami M (2013) Nursing ethical values and definitions: a literature review. Iran J Nurs Midwifery Res 18(1):1–8

Sheer B, Wong FKYM (2008) The development of advanced nursing practice globally. J Nurs Sch 40(3):204–211

Swift A, Twycross A (2020) Using ways of knowing in nursing to develop educational strategies that support knowledge mobilization. Peadiatr Neonatal Pain 2(4):139–147. https://doi.org/10.1002/pne2.12037

Throne S (2020) Rethinking carper's personal knowledge for 21st century nursing. Nurs Philos 21:e12307. https://doi.org/10.1111/nup.12307

Torrens C, Campbell P, Hoskins G, Strachan H, Wells M, Cunningham M, Bottone H, Polson R, Maxwell M (2020) Barriers and facilitators to the implementation of the advanced nurse practitioner role in primary care settings: a scoping review. Int J Nurs Stud 104:103443. https://doi.org/10.1016/j.ijnurstu.2019.103443. Epub 2019 Sep 27. PMID: 32120089

Tracy MF, O'Grady ET (eds.) (2019) Hamric and hanson's advanced practice nursing: an integrative approach, 6th ed. Elsevier. ISBN:978-0-323-44775-1

Wiener J (2016) A global perspective on advance practice nurses in primary care. https://ldi.upenn.edu/healthpolicysense/global-perspective-advance-practice-nurses-primary-care. Accessed 19 Dec 2019

Woo BFY, Zhou W, Lim TW, Tam WWS (2019) Practice patterns and role perception of advanced practice nurses: a nationwide cross-sectional study. J Nurs Manag 27:992–1004. https://doi.org/10.1111/jonm.12759

Xue Y, Ye Z, Brewer C, Spetz J (2016) Impact of state nurse practitioner scope-of-practice regulation on health care delivery: systematic review. Nurs Outlook 64(1):71–85. https://doi.org/10.1016/j.outlook.2015.08.005

Factors Influencing Perceptions

3

3.1 Introduction

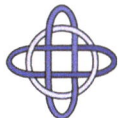

This chapter explores different factors that can influence your perceptions of the APN role and your role transition process. Perceptions are built upon one's current knowledge and beliefs. Understanding yourself as nurse, APN, student, family member, and recognizing your strengths are important steps towards success. This chapter provides insight and knowledge on the APN role and formation of your professional identity.

Exemplar

Bella is in her second year of her APN graduate education. The educational process has been demanding with many topics and processes that have been new to Bella. She has been feeling overwhelmed and inadequate; thus, she has been considering leaving the program and return to her nursing job where she was considered an expert with her oncology patients. Bella confided in another student, Ingrid, that she did not feel that she should become an APN. The two students sat to share their thoughts and fears about the APN role. Ingrid reminded Bella that as an oncology nurse expert Bella had confidence, courage, the ability to implement change, and believed she was supporting the role of nursing through her high-quality care she provided. They discussed how difficult the education process was concerning the change in knowledge in becoming the prescriber of the care and the emotions with feeling like a novice. Then they shared their curiosity on what it will be like when they graduated and were APNs in the workplace. Each decided to help each other to have the courage to continue and remind each other of the personal strengths they have to become APN.

© The Author(s), under exclusive license to Springer Nature Switzerland AG 2022   57
M. Kidner, *Successful Advanced Practice Nurse Role Transition*, Advanced
Practice in Nursing, https://doi.org/10.1007/978-3-030-53002-0_3

3.2   Definitions

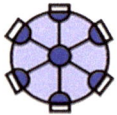

Barriers According to dictionary.com anything that restrains or obstructs progress, access is considered a barrier. In the context of this book, "barriers" are any challenges that can create difficulty for a generalist or specialist nurse acquiring the graduate-level advanced nursing education, role transition to APN, or implementing the role in the workplace.

Clinical leadership Clinical leadership is a complex and interrelated process of expert direct clinical practice, effective communication, effective interprofessional relationships, team working with empowerment, mentoring and influencing stakeholders towards common healthcare goals (Stanley and Stanley 2018). Clinical leadership includes the knowledge, skills to provide nursing care combined with the ability to communicate, mentor, advocate, educate, collaborate, and build trust relationships with all stakeholders. Clinical leadership usually is an informal role. A key component of clinical leadership is the lack of subordination between the clinical leader and the followers. Clinical leadership is often an informal role and develops as other watch the increased knowledge, skills, critical thinking, and patient care thereby developing trust and the desire to follow the APN.

Courage The mental or moral strength to try something new, persevere under difficulties, or withstand danger, fear, or challenges is courage. There are three types of courage: TRY Courage, TRUST Courage, and TELL Courage. Courageous workers take on more challenging projects, cope better with change, and speak up on important issues (Treasurer 2019).

Concept Analysis A "concept analysis" is a methodical and rigorous inquiry surrounding the concept's elements to promote clarity and enhance the understanding within nursing (Foley and Davis 2017).

Curiosity Curiosity is more than having an interest in a topic. Curiosity is a strong desire to know or learn something to reduce information gaps and cognitive uncertainty. In addition to the desire of obtaining knowledge, there is a sense that closing the information gap is possible and desirable regardless of extrinsic rewards (Pekrun 2019).

Self-perceptions A personal viewpoint of self (mental or physical attributes) that constitute the self. One's personal view of self may involve genuine self-knowledge or varying degrees of distortion (https://dictionary.apa.org/self-perception accessed 12/18/2021). There are several aspects of self-perceptions and each has unique aspects. In this book, self-concept and self-efficacy are components discussed.

3.3   Curiosity and Courage to Change

To be willing to endure a change, the person must first be curious about the possibilities and potential outcome the change may cause. Yet even before willingness there must be curiosity. There is research on curiosity (Pekrun 2019; Russell 2013). Curiosity often precedes motivation, which in turn results in people exploring new knowledge, skills, and behaviors (Russell 2013). The activity of curiosity contributes to expanding knowledge and skills for becoming an APN through enhancing creative and critical thinking/decision-making. The desire to want to learn and to be challenged is often because the person is curious about what future possibilities can occur once the new knowledge is implemented (Russell 2013). It is anticipated that your desire to obtain the student APN experiences of education and practice is partly because you are curious about how you will help and provide healthcare services to your future patients.

Being curious is an excellent attribute that drives inquiry and motivation. Intellectual curiosity can be fostered, engaged, or sustained through internal or external motivators. As you transition from student to APN remember inspiring intellectual curiosity in your patients can help them to seek new knowledge and behaviors for a healthier lifestyle and/or understanding your plans of their care.

According to the Merriam-Webster dictionary (https://www.merriam-webster.com/dictionary/courage), courage is the mental or moral strength to venture, persevere, and withstand danger, fear, or difficulty. APN education and the transition process to practice can be difficult at times. You will enhance your confidence in APN knowledge, skills, decisions, and leadership as you explore your professional identity (Haghighat et al. 2020). Being curious, asking questions, seeking knowledge and experiences, and having the courage to change will build your confidence and provide the foundation of your professional identity as an APN.

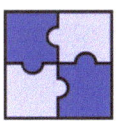

Write 1–2 statements concerning topics you are studying that you are curious about and what would like to explore to expand your knowledge.

_____
_____
_____
_____
_____

3.4   Looking at History

The APN role is relatively new. Have you ever been curious about how APN got started? It is meaningful to look at the past to fully appreciate the APN role development in your country and internationally. There are challenges and barriers to overcome during any change process. Implementing the APN role has been no different. Understanding the courage to change and paths others have taken around the world to pioneer and expand the APN role can provide you with insight and courage to continue to grow the APN role in your country.

Currently (in 2022) the international recognition of the APN role as a specific graduate degree program includes the CRNA, CNS, and NP roles. In chronological order of the development of these roles is CRNA then CNS then NP. Each has a unique past that started with an unmet healthcare need where nurses responded to fill the need.

3.4.1   The Courage and Vision of Role Developers

The discovery of ether as an anesthetic would impact the development of the APN role of the CRNA (ICN 2021 Guidelines on Advanced Practice Nursing Nurse Anesthetists). Surgeons realized the immense impact of ether to surgery and also realized that they could not be responsible for both the anesthesia and the surgery. As early as 1863 there has been documentation that nurses provided anesthesia for surgery (Tracy et al. 2019). Dr. William Worrall Mayo (who establishes the Mayo clinic) was among the first physicians to hire and formally train nurse anesthetists by early 1890s. Over the years, wars have driven the advancement and role of the CRNA as science, technology, and advanced skills requirements increased in anesthesiology changing the educational demands and requirements from specialized nursing to a postgraduate certificate to a masters' degree for the APN recognition (Tracy et al. 2019; ICN 2021). Ether was first used as an inhalation anesthetic was on October 16, 1846 by William T.G. Morton, a Boston (United States) dentist. Thus, the CRNA role has its beginning in the United States (Chang et al. 2015).

In 1923, a Winslow-Goldmark committee report in the United States wrote about the need for nursing clinical experts (Fulton et al. 2019). Francis Reiter used the term nurse-clinician in a 1943 speech which provided inspiration for Hildegard Peplau (McClelland et al. 2013). Hildegard Peplau set the paradigm of graduate education for advancing nursing and the development of the CNS role by developing the first master's degree program for psychiatric nursing (Drew 2014; Mayo et al. 2017). However, she did not stop there. Peplau was dedicated to the development of advanced nursing education, she is considered the "mother of the psychiatric nurse" through her revolutionary work in patient–nurse relationships, and personal work on professional boards impacting scope, regulation, and education nationally and internationally. The work and influence of Hildegard Peplau continue today and are valued by nurses and nursing organizations around the world. Her ideas have been incorporated into virtually every nursing specialty and into the practices of other healthcare professionals.

It is important to recognize that even the earliest visions (*Nursing for the Future* [E. L. Brown, 1948]) of the developing CNS role were to improve the nursing education for:

- Expert in clinical nursing knowledge and skills
- Providing advanced nursing skills and knowledge for direct patient care
- Possessing discriminative judgment
- Making a unique contribution to the prevention and treatment of illness
- Demonstrating clinical leadership
  - Improve nursing skills and develop new nursing skills
  - Teach and supervise other nurses and ancillary workers
  - Cooperate with other professions in planning for health at community, state, national, and international levels
  - Lead the delivery of care by others providing nursing care (Fulton 2020)

In addition, the desire for the CNS role was to be designed for the nurse to gain the professional competencies at a graduate level was an early role requirement (Fulton 2020).

Throughout the ages nurses have responded to the needs of other finding creative ways to provide the needed care. Evidence of such courageous caring was from 1893 to 1950 where Lillian Wald developed a nursing home visitation program that included education and medications to a poor New York City neighborhood. Although there was no formal training that led to a role development, these nurses used both regulatory and collaborative practices (Tracy et al. 2019; ICN 2021). Nurses responded to provide care to those in rural settings where there were no physicians, or populations which physicians did not want to provide care. Yet, the real design for the nurse practitioner came out of rural Colorado where the unmet healthcare needs were mothers and children unable to obtain healthcare due to their rural location (Tracy et al. 2019; ICN 2021).

In 1965 responding to the unmet needs in the United States concerning the care of mothers and children in the rural settings, Loretta Ford (an assistant professor) partnered with Dr. Henry Silver (a pediatrician) and initiated the Nurse Practitioner (NP) role (Keeling 2015). Dr. Ford reported that she had support from pediatricians, however lacked support from fellow nurses and nurse educators! The nurses felt Ford had overstepped the scope and role of the Registered Nurse (personal contact with Ford LC 2013, 2016). However, Dr. Ford persevered through the challenges and found ways to overcome barriers that led to the establishment of the NP role. The NP role in the USA started as a post-bachelor's certificate and evolved over time to the graduate level requirement. Internationally, the ICN endorses the graduate-level educational requirement. This nursing role is still meeting the unmet healthcare needs of millions of people worldwide.

3.4.2   Self as a Factor of Perception: Finding Strength Within

Understanding and self-review of self are essential (Michael 2019). The practice of a self-review enables people to play a part in their self-development, adaptation, and self-renewal (Bandura 2001; Michael 2019). Your belief in your capabilities to have control over your own functioning and over events that affect your life is your self-efficacy. As discussed in Chap. 2, Carper's personal way of knowing can provide a process to the awareness and effectiveness of self-reflection (Throne 2020). When one has a positive sense of self-efficacy, then it can provide the foundation for motivation, courage, well-being, and personal accomplishment (Lopez-Garrido 2020).

People's beliefs in their efficacy are developed by several sources of influence, including:

1. Mastery with experiences: Your ability to obtain knowledge and skills by hands-on experiences.
2. Vicarious experiences: Learning through discussions and case studies.
3. Social persuasion: Curiosity, discussions, and support from other APN students, instructors, and support people.
4. Emotional states: Impacted from internal and external factors.
5. A set of values and beliefs: Impacts how well one can execute a plan of action.
6. Determination, courage, and perseverance: How one overcomes obstacles that would interfere with goal attainment.

The most influential source on self-efficacy is the personal interpretation of one's previous performance, or when one has successfully accomplished a new challenge (Lopez-Garrido 2020). This is why honest self-review is meaningful to success in the APN role transition and professional identity process. High self-efficacy has been linked with numerous benefits to daily life, such as an improved ability to address adverse and stress events, incorporating healthy lifestyle habits, improved work performance/capacity, and higher educational achievement (Lopez-Garrido 2020). Yet, often our perception of self is inaccurate as we often underestimate our abilities, capabilities, and resilience.

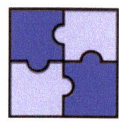

List at least three personal strengths you recognize within yourself:

_____
_____
_____
_____
_____

The development of your professional identity does not occur in a straight line. There will be gains and changes as you view and review your personal growth, self-accountability, self-resiliency, and confidence as you progress through your education towards APN (Cruess et al. 2019). Your personal habits and beliefs will impact your professional identity. The identity of APN includes the set of knowledge and practices that APNs do worldwide. Your professional identity includes the sharing of this set of APN knowledge, practices, global values, and ethics as APN that you identify as person and nurse (Gutierrez and Morais 2017). As you grow and transition through your education and clinical experiences, you will develop a sense of competence and confidence that is critical for a positive self-efficacy and for the growth of your APN professional identity.

3.4.3   Your Experiences and Personal factors

Although your clinical experiences are a central part of your formation of professional identity, there are also personal factors that impact the development of your professional identity as APN. Each of these factors impact your curiosity, courage, and self-efficacy.

These personal factors can include:

- Your perceived traditions of current workplace policy (such as caring for the poor in the emergency room or pediatric pain management).
- Your proficiency of required APN skills.
- Your advanced knowledge and ability to apply that knowledge in clinical settings.
- Your levels of confidence in deviating from workplace norms and culture when you know you are correct.
- Your past experiences as a nurse in providing care.
- Your past experiences in relationships to how you were respected by peers, staff, and physicians. (This determines the level of trust and integrity others have placed upon you.)
- Your perceived social norms of the workplace and nursing. This includes your courage, self-confidence, and self-resiliency to be an advocate when faced with a dilemma.
- Your ability to share and talk after significant events.
- Your personal value system, beliefs, and assumptions that guide your personal moral code and ethics.
- Your sense of belonging to your nursing role and workplace colleagues.
- Your desires for the future (will you be an advocate for others? What do you want to be doing in 3, 5, and 10 years from now?) (Barlow et al. 2018; Gutierrez and Morais 2017; Karanikola et al. 2018; Wald 2015: Walleck 1991).

3.4.4   Personal-Insight Learning Activity

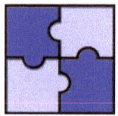

Review the list of personal factors, choose at least three and write how those factors currently impact your perception of who you are and the APN you will become.

_____
_____
_____
_____
_____
_____

Research on APN role transition and the experiences of the first year of APN practice have revealed a high level of personal feelings of APN role ambiguity with difficulty going from an expert general nurse to a novice APN (Barnes 2015; Faraz 2016; Owens 2019). Recognition of your strengths within and learning about the APN role, role transition, and professional identity can increase your success.

3.5   Role as a Factor of Perception

A "role" is a collection of connected specialized skills, knowledge, rights, behaviors, ethics, and standards held to be required to fulfill a social situation with expected behaviors of the profession (Owens 2019). The APN role is a unique advanced nursing role. The advanced skills range from complex care management to emergent care. The advanced knowledge of the APN includes advanced history and physical assessments, pharmacology, ordering and interpreting laboratory and diagnostics, differential diagnosing, process evaluation and design, enhanced clinical judgment and decisions, clinical leadership, utilization of systems management and change implementation. The particular scope of practice of an APN that is unique in nursing can include:

- the autonomy to admit/discharge a patient
- design and implement a treatment plan
- provide consultations
- order laboratory/diagnostics
- interpretations of exams and data
- determining diagnosis
- provide autonomous direct patient care

One may say that all levels of nursing can provide some aspects of the above activities. This is true. However, it is important to understand that the APN role is unique and provides benefit to the patient and workplace by *how* the APN implements these activities in a scope of practice. An APN uses clinical leadership through guidance, coaching, evidence-based practice, relationship building, and ethical decision-making blended together in all activities (Tracy et al. 2019). The APN's direct practice skill interacts with and informs all the other competencies. *It is an expectation that every APN embodies these competencies and seamlessly blends them into daily clinical practice* (Tracy et al. 2019).

However, it is prudent to recognize that these interwoven clinical leadership competencies develop over time and experience of the APN role. As you gain experience and through self-reflection with a structured process of role transition, you will gain confidence, self-efficacy, and professional identity as APN through the seamless blending of the APN competencies to practice at the top of your country's scope of practice.

The APN behaviors and ethics are the same as all nursing. The APN role can seem both exciting and overwhelming for students or new graduates to achieve. Yet, perceptions change over your course of APN education and role attainment. You will find that your perceptions and abilities (skills, knowledge, decisions, and leadership) improve with your curiosity, courage, and determination to become an APN.

3.6   Concept Analysis of Professional Identity

Professional identity includes the behaviors and activities of self and others in the same profession. The characteristics of professional identity include internalization of core values and beliefs of the profession and maintaining the ethics and values in the context of practice. Interestingly, the incorporation of one's professional ethics and values typically occurs after obtaining the required specialized knowledge and skills (Fitzgerald 2020).

APNs are unique within the nursing profession. APNs obtain:

1. An advanced body of nursing knowledge based on evidence on both scientific and nursing research. APN nursing education is based on nursing theories and healthcare.
2. A process to use self-reflection of one's own practice to contribute to healthcare practices and develop a positive professional identity with a strong nursing ethic base.
3. An advanced and unique set of skills to fulfill the role based on the country's need.
4. The ability to make critical decisions maintaining nursing ethics in settings of uncertainty and complexity.
5. A continuation of growing the body of knowledge and using evidence-based practice (EBP) to improve processes and outcomes.

6. A community of nursing professionals who perform oversight and monitoring of professional practice.
7. Positive interactions and relationship building with all stakeholders.
8. Education on leadership in clinical and formal roles.

3.6.1   What Is a Concept Analysis?

The concept analysis has become a frequent technique in nursing research (Foley and Davis 2017; Rodgers et al. 2018). This research process requires critical appraisal of literature data concerning all aspects of the topic being explored (the "concept") to clarify and define the concept for future model or theory development. A "concept" is a thought, or idea, concerning a particular topic or process. Concepts are foundational building blocks of thoughts and beliefs leading to categorization, inference, and learning (https://www.merriam-webster.com/dictionary/concept; Margolis et al. 2021). Within nursing research, a concept is an abstract idea the researcher wants to pursue to clarify and define so that it will become a building block of a bigger spectrum (Foley and Davis 2017). The bigger spectrum of collected building blocks can become a theory. Thus, a "concept analysis" is a methodical and rigorous inquiry surrounding the concept's elements to promote clarity and enhance the understanding within nursing (Foley and Davis 2017).

Concept analysis with research rigor should clearly state the framework in which the analysis used to discover new knowledge and attributes that will lead to the operationalization of the concept (Rodgers et al. 2018). The following list includes several common nursing concept analyses frameworks:

- Wilson method (Walker and Avant 2011)
- Evolutionary method (Rodgers 2000)
- Principle-based method (Morse et al. 1996)
- Hybrid method (Schwartz-Barcott and Kim 2000)
- Concept clarification (Norris 1982)
- Dimensional analysis (Schatzman and Strauss 1973; Bowers 2021)

This book uses two concept analyses to help explore the process a nurse goes through to become an APN: professional identity and role transition. Both researchers used the Walker and Avant's Wilson methodology (Walker and Avant 2011) for the exploration of the concepts. This methodology provides the research-specific steps to evaluate a concept, determine common themes, and provide specific case studies to clarify the concept. The research steps in the Wilson Method (Walker and Avant 2011) include:

- A comprehensive literature search on all aspects concerning the concept
- Definitions
- Defining attributes

- Model case
- Borderline case
- Contrary case
- Consequences
- Antecedents
- Empirical referents
- Discussion
- Conclusions

For the purposes of this book, the aspects of a concept analysis that are most relevant to understand the concept and implications in clinical practice will be discussed. The three aspects of a concept analysis of the two concepts (professional identity and role transition) that will be discussed are:

- Defining attributes
- Antecedents
- Consequences

3.6.2   Professional Identity Concept Analysis Attributes

A defining attribute is **an aspect** (a time or process) **that is highly characteristic of the concept** (Walker and Avant 2011). The Fitzgerald concept analysis of professional identity has five defining attributes. They are actions and behaviors; knowledge and skills; values, beliefs and ethics; context and socialization; and group and personal identity (Fitzgerald 2020). Let us examine each attribute:

1. **Actions and Behaviors**
   Actions and behaviors of a profession are strongly linked to identifying with that profession (Fitzgerald 2020). The APN professional identity is derived from what APNs see other APNs do; in essence the behaviors and activities of APNs become what we identify as our APN profession. When actions and tasks being performed are what are anticipated of the APN role, then the attachment to APN professional identity is greater. The APN's actions and behavior are embedded in our nursing ethics, values, and process of assessment, planning, implementation, and evaluation.
2. **Knowledge and Skills**
   When the common knowledge and skills are required for the professional role and the knowledge and skills support the values of the profession within the social context, then they become the foundation of professionalism (Fitzgerald 2020). Knowledge and skills separate the levels of nursing from general, specialized, and advanced practice. The professional self requires that you integrate the knowledge, theories, frameworks, expertise, experience, and professionalism as key components of knowledge and skills applied to APN practice.

3. **Values, Beliefs, and Ethics**

   The most cited attributes of a profession are commonly held values, beliefs, and ethics of that profession (Fitzgerald 2020). Individuals typically incorporate the professional values and ethics after they have confidence in the required knowledge and skills. Yet knowledge and skills alone do not make the profession. Nursing professionalism, and professional identity, includes the embodiment of the code of ethics, understanding social values, recognizing the context and local culture, and having members who are motivated by altruism and committed to the profession. Many nurses find meaning to their profession through the professional values that makes the nursing profession unique.

4. **Context and Socialization**

   Context and socialization support occurs when a person identifies with a group of people in the same role, then self-identification as a member of the role is strengthened (Fitzgerald 2020). A significant aspect of a positive professional identity is being a member of the profession and accepting the responsibilities of the role to society and all stakeholders. Context includes self-regulation and self-identification of the role's responsibilities with enhanced accountability and authority in the setting of local political, cultural, and historical realities that surround them. As APNs provide high-quality, safe, patient-centered care, society recognizes the importance of the APN role which subsequently increases professional identity.

5. **Group and Personal Identity**

   Recognition by society and professional associations of each member within the group creates group identity which directly enhances personal identity to the profession (Fitzgerald 2020). The interdisciplinary work of APNs fosters a group identity in which nurses are influenced by and still differentiated from others that collaborate in patient care. Consistent professional actions using a specialized set of knowledge and skills combined with decisions made with integrity enhances attachment to a group/role. The attachment to a group directly impacts professional identity formation.

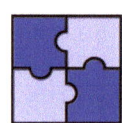

Review the five defining attributes of professional identity. Choose 1–2 attributes that are particularly meaningful to you and write how the attributes can help clarify your professional identity formation.

_____

_____

_____

_____

_____

_____

3.6.3   Concept Antecedents

Antecedents are events, or accomplishments, that must be achieved **before** the concept can be understood and personally incorporated (Walker and Avant 2011, p. 167). The primary antecedents for nursing professional identity by the Fitzgerald (2020) concept analysis is the completion of the educational degree, certification (or both) and recognizing the proper knowledge and skills to work within the profession. For a strong, positive nursing professional identity, Fitzgerald reported the following antecedents are required for the development of a strong professional identity:

- Autonomy (the ability and authority to provide healthcare without supervision)
- Responsibility (to accept the consequences of actions providing advanced nursing)
- Confidence (a personal positive self-confidence in the required skills and knowledge of APN practice)
- Clinical judgment (the ability to combine theory, knowledge, and clinical practice to make correct diagnosis and decisions)
- Ability to collaborate with others (enhanced team working abilities)
- Supportive organizational structure (where APN nursing fits into the workplace hierarchy)
- Proper resources (have same supplies and support as physicians)

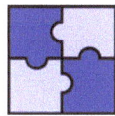

Review the antecedents of professional antecedents, which ones do you use already?

_____

_____

3.6.4   Concept Consequences

Consequences are the events that result from occurrence of the concept; they are the outcomes on the concept (Walker and Avant 2011, p. 167). Fitzgerald (2020) reports consequences for both a strong professional identity and a weak professional identity:

Strong Professional Identity Consequences

- Higher immunity to stress
- Enhanced self-confidence
- Positive attitudes
- Higher job satisfaction

- Feelings of achievement
- Better patient safety outcomes
- Improved patient outcomes
- Increased satisfaction with practice and role
- Improved retention (staying in the APN role and profession)

Weak Professional Identity Consequences

- Superficial commitment to the profession
- Poor quality of nursing
- Values dissonance
- Increased personal stress
- Decreased self-confidence
- Poor decision-making ability
- Allowing others to define the profession

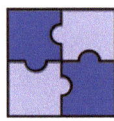

Review the potential consequences of professional identity formation and choose the ones you want to obtain. Are there antecedents that will impact your acquisition of your chosen consequences?

_____
_____
_____

As you go through this book, you will gain knowledge and complete activities that will support a positive professional identity acquisition. Being curious of the APN role that is being implemented worldwide, gaining knowledge of the impacts APNs are having on patient care and access to high-quality healthcare worldwide, and developing courage to implement your role will create a strong, positive attachment to the APN profession: your professional identity.

Conclusion of Professional Identity Concept Analysis

The evolution of your nursing career is a process that will involve the shaping and reshaping of your professional identity. Your self-concept and professional identity are strengthened through the identification with others through sense of shared group membership (group and personal identity with context and socialization). Your identification with other APNs may be simply by joining a local or national APN association. However, if you live remotely or there are very few APNs, you will need to be creative in developing a connection for group identity. APN actions and behaviors; knowledge and skills; and values, beliefs, and ethics are acquired through your graduate education and clinical practice sites.

Activities for APNs Working in Clinical Sites with Few APNs
1. Develop a positive trust relationship with a physician
2. Verify the description of the APN role is clearly written and shared in the workplace
3. Support and share about the APN role to your stakeholders
4. Offer to lead a team or project
5. Support and publicly advocate for all nursing roles (this can decrease jealousy within nursing roles)

3.7 Anticipate and Plan Role Impact on Personal Decisions

As you review different perception points of the APN role (self, role, and professional identity), it is important to anticipate and determine your action for potential scenarios. To anticipate is to be curious, to plan is to self-reflect and consider self-efficacy, and to act is to be courageous. The impact of your actions and behavior is the evolutionary process of your professional identity formation.

A planned, structured process for professional identity review requires time to reflect on past clinical complex decisions, skills, and ethics you have encountered plus the formation of a personal set of values that are habitual in times of stress and ethical within an academic setting that is organized and guided by self-introspection and key stakeholders (Gutierrez and Morais 2017; Wald 2015; Poorchangizi 2019; Pullen 2021). A highly effective practice is a formal post-clinical discussion with a specific intent on helping students assess the clinical experience and form an opinion or decision. If your graduate education offers post-clinical discussions, be an active participant. If your education program does not offer this practice, you may suggest a trial of post-clinical discussions to help students learn from each other and discuss professional identity in a structured process.

Exemplar
Thomas is in his fifth rotation in his APN graduate program and is an emergency room (ER) rotation. A mother brings in a 3-year-old child who fell out of a tree and fractured her femur. The child and mother are dirty, wearing thin, old, and tattered clothing yet interact in a caring way towards each other. The child is not crying while lying in the bed. The X-ray reveals a displaced, commuted fracture just below the femur head. Thomas asked his preceptor if he could medicate the child and he was told, "No, only medicate pediatric patients if they cry." The preceptor then told Thomas to ignore the child and mother and give his attention to other "critical and worthy" patients as the ER was very busy that day. Thomas is confused because his preceptor is an APN in the emergency room and she is well thought of by the staff and hospital leadership. Thomas now has a dilemma when comparing his own ethics and understanding of evidence-based practices concerning pediatric pain response and the type of injury versus the response of a person who is deemed, "an expert" APN. There is a disconnect.

How Thomas works through this ethical dilemma will become part of his foundation of his professional identity as APN. Should he explain the best practices on evaluations and treatment of pediatric trauma patients, or should he ignore the child and follow his preceptor incorporating her ethics into his paradigm and professional identity? Thus, it is important to understand the process on forming an identity. There are two options:

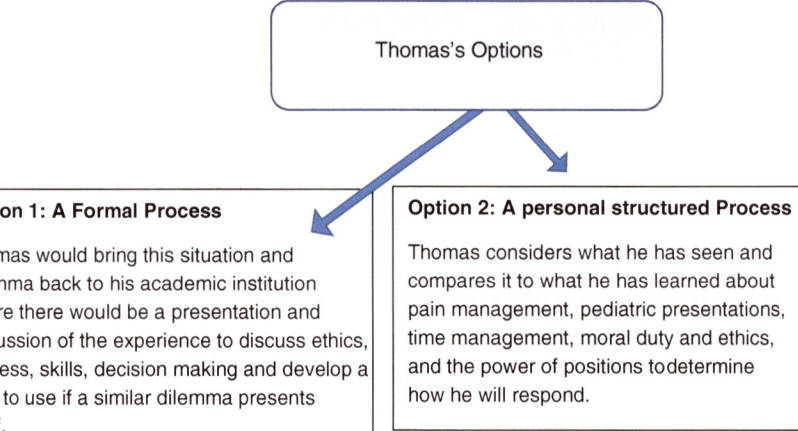

The formal, or structured, process involving instructors and students allows for a greater sharing of experiences, ethics, and decision-making. Many students with different experiences can help their peers through sharing and discussions (Bandura 2018). Yet, you can be successful in shaping your ethics, integrity, and personal value system by completing a structured process of dilemma evaluation and response. The first step in success is recognizing the need for a process to review, discuss, and determine future responses of personal and healthcare dilemmas. A personal structured process involves self-reflective practice.

3.7.1 Self-Reflection

Using self-reflection, you will construct your own learning within your paradigm based on your experiences, competencies, knowledge, and what you believe is right (Helberget et al. 2021). Reflection is a key phenomenon for your development into an APN role because you will have many complex and unpredictable situations arising in your clinical practice. The practice self-reflection will aid in your creative and critical decisions. Conflict, disagreement, and unexpected outcomes drive learning—even if the conflict is within yourself (Kolb and Kolb 2006). Learning and knowledge acquisition occur from these resolutions of conflict, disagreements, and unexpected outcomes (Kolb and Kolb 2006).

According to David Kolb's theory (1984), learning is a process in which competence is formed through the transformation of experience in four stages (Helberget et al. 2021).

1. You experience a given situation.
2. You reflect on the experiences and what it meant to you.
3. Using your reflective observations, you then generalize or formalize the learning outcomes of your experience into abstract thoughts and plans.
4. Later, this competence can be tested in new contexts.

When do you use self-reflection?

1. **Before an action or decision**: Consider the situation in advance to become more prepared for what is going to happen.
2. **During an action or decision:** When you handle an unexpected or difficult situation well, think about your actions and decisions that allowed you to be flexible and overcome the unexpected.
3. **After an action or decision:** Look back on the situation and critically appraise what went well, what did not go as expected, why did the situation unfold like it did, and what will you do in the future.

Self-reflection will be an asset to your APN role transition and the development of your own clinical practice. Through repeated exposure to situations and clinical decisions lead to a refinement of your earlier thoughts and ideas. Your knowledge acquisition and ability to respond to future similar events are increased if you write your self-reflections down in a journal.

Note to Students

If your school has a formal post-clinical process to discuss your clinical experiences, then use this time to share clinical dilemmas, or traumatic experiences to gain a stronger insight and decisions on how you will respond in the future.

If your school does not have a post-clinical time/process to discuss your experiences, then you can ask to set time in your didactic studies, or an online discussion board, or an instructor-led student forum to allow discussions on these complex clinical experiences. Group discussions can have a rich sharing of emotions, thoughts, ethics, assumptions, and knowledge that can drive decisions for future responses. Understanding other peoples' point of view is critical to a strong personal ethical framework.

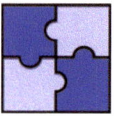

Activity For this activity you will need to choose one negative experience and one positive experience from your past nursing experience.

Choose an experience in the workplace where you observed something, or heard a discussion, that created uncertainty related to your ideas of professional nursing behavior (*a negative experience*). Describe the experience and determine what could have been done to improve the outcome of that experience.

A *negative experience* review will provide ideas how to improve and not repeat the same process that led to a negative outcome.

_____
_____
_____
_____
_____
_____
_____

Choose an experience in which you saw a peer complete an activity or discussion with expertise and integrity that you still hold it true and at a level you strive for daily (a positive experience). Determine the actions that you could repeat for a similar positive outcome.

A *positive experience* review provides a model, or steps to take to repeat positive outcomes in a similar situation.

_____
_____
_____
_____
_____
_____

3.8   Understand Context as Barrier or as Potential to Improve Relationships

Developing professional identity and a self-concept construction is particularly vulnerable during times of stress (Bentley et al. 2019; Emery et al. 2018; Wood and Olivier 2004). Role stress from traumatic events (such as a poor performance, missed diagnosis, a missed skill, or receiving negative feedback) can impact self-concept and professional identity formation. Most APNs will experience a negative event that occurred from a knowledge or process barrier.

Many barriers can block your ability to use your full scope of practice as APN. Barriers can cause you role transition stress. People placing clinical practice barriers for you to overcome typically result from simple lack of knowledge to overt passive aggressive acts. It is imperative to understand possible barriers so that you can recognize barriers and develop skills to overcome the stressful events. Below are six common barriers that can impact the implementation of the role to clinical practice and thus your role transition process from general nursing to APN. Barriers are discussed in greater detail in Chap. 7 with actions you can do to decrease workplace barriers.

1. **Role ambiguity.** Role ambiguity can also occur when the APN and the other stakeholders hold different viewpoints and understanding of the role responsibility, accountability, and authority (Jones 2014). Different viewpoints can be related to the misunderstanding of the scope of practice in your country (remember scope of practice is usually determined on a country/state level and not workplace). When there is a poor knowledge of the APN role, or a poor job description, or when formal leadership, other healthcare providers, and policy decision makers do not have a clear understanding of the scope of practice then misunderstandings and role ambiguity occur (Gutierrez and Morais 2017; Karanikola et al. 2018; Klein et al. 2020; Thompson 2019; Vaismoradi et al. 2011). APNs can receive role ambiguity barriers from:
   (a) Patients and patient's family members
   (b) Physicians and hospital staff
   (c) Supervisors and senior leadership
   (d) Friends and APN's family members
   (e) Stakeholders and government officials
   (f) The society in general
2. **Failure to complete introspective self-exploration.** To obtain a strong sense of self within the new nursing role as APN one must spend time on introspective self-review and exploration (Cruess et al. 2019; Hernandez et al. 2017; MacLellan et al. 2015). It is essential to understand yourself as person and as nurse to develop a strong self-concept and professional identity (Bell and Leite 2016). Critical and creative thinking with ethical decision-making processes are embedded within your personal values, beliefs, attitudes, and past experiences (Laukkonen and Slagter 2021; Vinje and Mittelmark 2008; Walleck 1991).
3. **Vertical discounting**. This occurs when a subordinate, or supervisor, refuses to recognize your full scope of practice. Vertical discounting often occurs when generalist or specialist nursing staff holds a negative view of the APN role and feels the role has moved away from traditional nursing and therefore refuse to follow the prescribed care written by the APN (Anderson et al. 2020). Vertical discounting can also occur from a formal supervisor or physician that purposefully refuse to allow the APN to provide care in the full scope of practice. This discounting is intentional, and the result can undermine the APN's authority to prescribe treatment plans.
4. **Lateral Othering**. Lateral othering occurs when there is negative behavior (ambivalence, the silent treatment, bullying, or passive aggressive behavior) among APNs (Anderson et al. 2020). This type of barrier comes from someone with your same

level of responsibility, accountability, and authority: one APN to another APN. Lateral othering is detrimental to one's confidence and successful transition.

5. **Work-Family imbalance**. When a person spends too much time at work (or in school) an imbalance between work/school requirements and family needs can occur. Work-family imbalance results in increased emotional stress and decreased work engagement (Klein et al. 2020). This imbalance can be caused by the family's feelings of abandonment related to time requirements of a graduate program and work, or feelings of anger and fear as there is a change in family income dynamics. Overcoming work-balance barriers requires support and discussions with your family to develop a mutually agreed plan. This plan requires an open discussion, plus recognition that it is healthy to have a well-balanced life between work, family, and relaxation.

6. **Shortage of resources**. To be an effective APN, you will need to have resources (equipment, staff, supplies, and funding). The APN should receive the same supplies and resources as the physician within the same workplace. Shortages of resources include all aspects that can impede your APN role implementation in your workplace. Problems can arise when there are shortages in appropriate accommodations, nursing staff, appropriate funding, administrative support (including technology), and resources for research and education (Jones 2014; Woo et al. 2019). These shortages can impact patient care, professional development, and personal morale (Jones 2014). Organizational structure, workplace culture, public opinion, and social support (such as the importance of the nursing role, women, or other disparities that can be aimed at nursing and APN) can directly impact the availability of resources (Jones 2014; ten Hoeve et al. 2013; Sheer and Wong 2008).

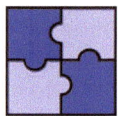

Discussion scenario Diana is a new APN graduate beginning her first job as an APN. She has 15 years of experience as a nurse before entering graduate school and was considered an expert in her internal medicine department. She feels well prepared from her APN education. When Diana begins her new job, she finds out that she does not have an office or personal space. The physician providers each have a personal office. She is also informed that she does not have any staff support to help bring her patients to the exam room and take the vital signs. She was informed that as a nurse she would be able to perform all the duties of nursing plus her APN role. Diana then inquires whether she is given more time to see patients as she will have added responsibilities in preparing the clinical patients for the visits. She is informed that she was hired as an APN provider and is expected to see the same number of patients per day as the physicians.

What are the potential barriers to Diana's successful APN role?

_____
_____
_____

In your opinion, how should Diana respond to her predicament?

_____
_____
_____

What can you do to prevent a similar scenario from happening to you?

_____
_____
_____

3.9   Self as Clinical Leader Perspective

A leader is a person who can maximize the efforts of others through positive social influence to achieve a mutually agreed goal (Kidner 2019). APNs, by virtue of their education, clinical expertise, and position in healthcare are seen as leaders. You may not have considered yourself in a leadership role, or yourself as a clinical leader.

Leadership is an internationally accepted component of APN (ICN 2020). Clinical expertise and the impact in leading the delivery of nursing care by others are core to several dimensions of the practicing APN that contributes to the view of the APN role as advanced nursing. Internationally, culture, sociopolitical status (health policies deployment and regulation), and leadership education impact the capacity of informal and formal APN roles (Lamb et al. 2018).

The increasing complexity and chaos of the world with political, social, and health issues have added to the unpredictable and dynamic environment in which APNs work. Such environments require healthcare professionals to demonstrate effective clinical leadership. Experienced formal and informal nurse leaders can help new leaders navigate the leadership process (Bove and Scott 2021).

Clinical leadership is a learned process. The process starts with understanding self. Chapters 5 and 6 will provide you with activities to build your personal set of values, vision, and mission to allow you to recognize your innate leadership. The sequel to this book is focused on clinical leadership. To continue to develop your clinical leadership skills and knowledge, you can:

- Listen intently to others
- Build positive and productive relationships (learn to respond to incivility and passive aggression)
- Show an authentic interest in the lives and professional development of staff
- Become highly competent with skills and knowledge for the patients you care for

- Set an example of intellectual integrity
- Create opportunities for shared decision-making
- Role model the nursing ethics
- Learn to delegate to others through your mentorship
- Offer honest feedback
- Empathize with others to help them overcome challenges (Bove and Scott 2021; Kidner 2019)

Leadership can be in the form of a formal role as a team leader, project lead, unit manager, or a member of a board. Or your leadership can be informal, and you lead through example and mentorship to others. Your informal leadership is your clinical leadership.

As an APN student it is beneficial to recognize that many of your current habits of behavior are already good leadership behaviors. You inspire, mentor, guide and support patients, staff, families, and others through your acts of nursing practice. As you work through your role transition, self-reflection, and find your courage to make a difference, your informal clinical leadership skills will increase. Becoming a "leader" is simply finding your positive social influences that you can apply to help maximize the efforts of others to achieve a mutually agreed goal (Kidner 2019).

What is the difference between attributes of clinical leader and informal leader?

"Informal Clinical Leadership"
An informal leader is a person who, by virtue of how he or she is perceived by others, is seen as worthy of paying attention to, or followed because that person evokes respect, confidence, and trust in others. The ability for an informal leader to inspire others to their maximum effort rests on the ability of that person and not a formal position they may hold.

What do you need to be an informal leader?
Credibility: You need to be knowledgeable, believable, and rational.

Integrity: You need to treat everyone with respect, assuming positive intent in others even when you disagree, communicating clearly and honestly, giving constructive feedback when necessary, listening carefully, and helping others to become their best.

Helping others: You need to help others on your team to learn and grow through mentoring and coaching.

(Bacal n.d. accessed 4 Feb 2020; Katz 2018; Kidner 2019)

As APN you will impact your stakeholders through your clinical leadership. Below are some aspects of the work environment you can impact with good informal clinical leadership skills and knowledge.

- High self and employee work satisfaction (job satisfaction, work engagement, decreased turnover).
- Improved work environment factors (role support, addressing negative behaviors, group relationships).

- Improved health and well-being of self and staff (emotional and physical stress of work).
- High-quality performance of self and others (job performance, knowledge sharing, creativity, feedback, mentorships).

3.10   Summary

This chapter provides the opportunity to explore different factors that can influence your perceptions of the APN role and your role transition process. Perceptions are built upon one's current knowledge and beliefs. This chapter provides insight and knowledge on the APN role and professional identity formation through discussions on:

- The influence of curiosity and courage has on your ability to increase your engagement to your APN education experiences.
- The influence of yourself as a factor of perception and the importance of recognizing your strengths as a person, nurse, and APN student.
- The influence of the APN role as a factor of personal perception of your future.
- Exploring the concept of professional identity through a concept analysis.
- Formal and informal review of experiences that will help you anticipate and plan responses.
- Recognition that there are barriers that have the potential to impact your perception of the APN role and yourself as an APN. These barriers can be used as ways to develop improved trust relationships.
- Recognition that the role of clinical leader is innately part of being an APN.

References

Anderson H, Birks Y, Adamson J (2020) Exploring the relationship between nursing identity and advanced nursing practice: an ethnographic study. J Clin Nurs 29:1195–1208. https://doi.org/10.1111/jocn.15155

Bacal R (n.d.) Leadership development for informal leaders. In: Leadership today. http://leadertoday.org/articles/developinformalleaders.htm. Accessed 4 Feb 2020

Bandura A (2001) Social cognitive theory: an agentic perspective. Annu Rev Psychol 52:1–26. https://doi.org/10.1146/annurev.psych.52.1.1

Bandura A (2018) Toward a psychology of human agency: pathways and reflections. Perspect Psychol Sci 13(2):130–136. https://doi.org/10.1177/1745691617699280

Barlow NA, Hargreaves J, Gillibrand W (2018) Nurses' contributions to the resolution of ethical dilemmas in practice. Nurs Ethics 25(2):230–242. https://doi.org/10.1177/0969733017703700

Barnes H (2015) Nurse practitioner role transition: a concept analysis, Nursing Forum 50(3):137–146

Bell D, Leite A (2016) Experiential self-understanding. Int J Psychoanal 97(2):305–332. https://doi.org/10.1111/1745-8315.12365. Epub 2016 Jan 25. PMID: 26804793

Bentley SV, Peters K, Haslam SA, Greenaway KH (2019) Construction at work: multiple identities scaffold professional identity development in academia. Front Psychol 10:628. https://doi.org/10.3389/fpsyg.2019.00628

Bove LA, Scott M (2021) Advice for aspiring nurse leaders. Nursing 51(3):44–47. https://doi.org/10.1097/01.NURSE.0000733952.19882.55

Bowers BJ, Schatzman L (2021) Dimensional analysis in developing grounded theory, 2nd edition. 2021. Imprint Routledge. eBook ISBN: 9781315169170

The Brown Report, AJN (1948) Am J Nurs 48(12):736–742

Chang CY, Goldstein E, Agarwal N, Swan KG (2015) Ether in the developing world: rethinking an abandoned agent. BMC Anesthesiol 15:149. https://doi.org/10.1186/s12871-015-0128-3. PMID: 26475128; PMCID: PMC4608178

Cruess S, Cruess R, Steinert Y (2019) Supporting the development of professional identity: general principles. Med Teach 41(6):641–649. https://doi.org/10.1080/0142159X.2018.1536260

Drew B (2014) The evolution of the role of the psychiatric mental health advanced practice registered nurse in the United States. Arch Psychiatr Nurs 28(5):298–300

Emery L, Gardner W, Carswell K, Finkel E (2018) You can't see the real me: attachment avoidance, self-verification, and self-concept clarity. Personal Soc Psychol Bull 44(8):1133–1146. https://doi.org/10.1177/0146167218760799

Faraz A (2016) Novice Nurse Practitioner Workforce transition into primary care: a literature review. West J Nurs Res 38(11):1531–1545. https://doi.org/10.1177/0193945916649587

Fitzgerald A (2020) Professional identity: a concept analysis. Nurs Forum 55:447–472. https://doi.org/10.1111/nuf.12450

Foley A, Davis A (2017) A guide to concept analysis. Clin Nurse Spec 31(2):70–73. https://doi.org/10.1097/NUR.0000000000000277

Ford LC (2013) Personal communication at the willow ceremony, University of Wyoming School of Nursing

Ford LC (2016) Personal communication. AANP National Conference

Fulton J (2020) Evolution of the clinical nurse specialist role and practice in the United States. In: Fulton JS, Goudreau KA, Swartzell KL (eds) Foundations of clinical nurse specialist practice. Springer Publishing Company, New York

Fulton S, Mayo A, Walker J, Urden L (2019) Description of work processes used by clinical nurse specialists to improve patient outcomes. Nurs Outlook 67(5):511–522. https://doi.org/10.1016/j.outlook.2019.03.001

Gutierrez MGR, Morais SCRV (2017) Systematization of nursing care in the formation of professional identity. Rev Bras Enferm 70(2):436—442. https://doi.org/10.1590/0034-7167-2016-0515

Haghighat S, Borhani F, Ranjbar H (2020) Is there a relationship between moral competencies and the formation of professional identity among nursing students? BMC Nurs 19:49. https://doi.org/10.1186/s12912-020-00440-y

Helberget LK, Aasen ME, Dahlborg E (2021) Learning about user participation among nursing students: a qualitative study. Nurse Educ Today 98:104660. https://doi.org/10.1016/j.nedt.2020.104660

Hernandez PR, Bloodhart B, Barnes RT, Adam AS, Clinton SM, Pollack I et al (2017) Promoting professional identity, motivation, and persistence: benefits of an informal mentoring program for female undergraduate students. PLoS One 12(11):e0187531. https://doi.org/10.1371/journal.pone.0187531

International Council of Nursing Guidelines on Advanced Practice Nursing 2020. Geneva. 2020. https://www.icn.ch/system/files/documents/2020-04/ICN_APN%20Report_EN_WEB.pdf. Accessed 17 April 2020

International Council of Nurses Guidelines on Advanced Practice Nursing Nurse Anesthetists 2021. Geneva. 2021. https://www.icn.ch/system/files/2021-07/ICN_Nurse-Anaesthetist-Report_EN_WEB.pdf. Accessed 18 April 2022

Jones ML (2014) Role development and effective practice in specialist and advanced practice roles in acute hospital settings: systematic review and meta-synthesis. J Adv Nurs 49(2):191–209

Karanikola M, Doulougeri K, Koutrouba A, Giannalopoulou M, Papathanassoglou EDE (2018) A phenomenological investigation of the interplay among professional wort appraisal, self-esteem and self-perception in nurses: the revelation of an internal and external criteria system. Front Psychol 9:1805. https://doi.org/10.3389/fpsyg.2018.01805

Katz H (2018) Informal leadership: leading without authority. https://medium.com/@harry_katz/informal-leadership-leading-without-authority-6373ff4e0a51. (Updated 9 Sept). Accessed 4 Feb 2020

Keeling AW (2015) Historical perspectives on an expanded role for nursing. Online J Issues Nurs 29(20):2. http://ojin.nursingworld.org/MainMenuCategories/ANAMarketplace/ANAPeriodicals/OJIN/TableofContents/Vol-20-2015/No2-May-2015/Historical-Perspectives-Expanded-Role-Nursing.html. Accessed 27 Apr 2020

Kidner M (2019) APN role transition with LEAP leadership. Copyright of unpublished works. TXu 2-166-138. The United States Copyright Office

Klein CJ, Weinzimmer LG, Lizer M, Colling M, Pierce L, Dalstrom M (2020) Exploring burnout and job stressors among advanced practice providers. Nurs Outlook 68(2):145–154. https://doi.org/10.1016/j.outlook.2019.09.005

Kolb A, Kolb D (2006) Learning styles and learning spaces: a review of the multidisciplinary application of experiential learning theory in higher education. Learning styles and learning: a key to meeting the accountability demands in education, pp 45–91

Lamb A, Martin-Misner R, Bryant-Lukosius D, Latimer M (2018) Describing the leadership capabilities of advanced practice nurses using a qualitative descriptive study. Nurs Open 5:400–413. https://doi.org/10.1002/nop2.150

Laukkonen RE, Slagter HA (2021) From many to (n)one: meditation and the plasticity of the predictive mind. Neurosci Biobehav Rev 128:199–217. https://doi.org/10.1016/j.neubiorev.2021.06.021. Epub 2021 Jun 14. PMID: 34139248

Lopez-Garrido G (2020) Self-efficacy theory. https://www.simplypsychology.org/self-efficacy.html published Aug 09, 2020. Accessed 16 Jun 2021

MacLellan L, Levett-Jones T, Higgins I (2015) Nurse practitioner role transition: a concept analysis. J Am Assoc Nurse Pract 27:389–397. https://doi.org/10.1002/2327-6924.12165

Margolis E, Laurence S (2021) "Concepts", The Stanford encyclopedia of philosophy (Spring 2021 Edition). In: Zalta EN (ed) https://plato.stanford.edu/archives/spr2021/entries/concepts/. Accessed 18 Jul 2021

Mayo AN et al (2017) The advanced practice clinical nurse specialist. Nurs Adm Q 41(1):70–76. https://doi.org/10.1097/NAQ.0000000000000201

McClelland M, McCoy MA, Burson R (2013) Clinical nurse specialist: then, now and future of the profession. Clinical Nurse Specialist 96–102. https://doi.org/10.1097/NUR.0b013e3182819154

Michael MT (2019) Self-insight. Int J Psychoanal 100(4):693–710. https://doi.org/10.1080/00207578.2019.1577111. PMID: 33952149

Morse JM, Mitcham C, Hupcey JE, Cerdas M (1996) Criteria for concept evaluation. J Adv Nurs 24(2):385–390. https://doi.org/10.1046/j.1365-2648.1996.18022.x

Norris, Catherine M (1982) Concept clarification in nursing/edited by Catherine M. Norris. Rockville, Md: Aspen Systems Corp. Print

Owen RA (2019) Nurse practitioner role transition and identity development in rural health settings: a scoping review. Nurs Educ Perspect 40(3):157–161. https://doi.org/10.1097/01.NEP.0000000000000455

Pekrun R (2019) The murky distinction between curiosity and interest: state of the art and future prospects. Educ Psychol Rev 31:905–914. https://doi.org/10.1007/s10648-019-09512-1

Poorchangizi B, Borhani F, Abbsazadeh A, Mirzaee M, Farokhzadian J (2019) Professional values of nurses and nursing students: a comparative study. BMC Medical Education 19:438. https://doi.org/10.1186/s12909-019-187-2

Pullen R (2021) Profession identity in nursing practice. Nursing made Incredibly easy. https://doi.org/10.1097/01.NME.0000732012.99855.78

Rodgers BL. Knafl KA (2000) concept development in nursing. Foundation, Techniques and Applications. 2nd Edition, Saunders, Philadelphia.

Rodgers BL, Jacelon CS, Knafl KA (2018) Concept analysis and the advance of nursing knowledge: state of the science. J Nurs Scholarsh 50(4):451–459. https://doi.org/10.1111/jnu.12386

Russell BH (2013) Intellectual curiosity: a principle-based concept analysis. ANS Adv Nurs Sci 36(2):94–105. https://doi.org/10.1097/ANS.0b013e3182901f74. PMID: 23644262

Schatzman L, Strauss AL (1973) Field research: Strategies for a natural sociology. Englewood Cliffs, N.J: Prentice-Hall

Schwartz-Barcott D, Kim (2000) An expansion and elaboration of the hybrid model of concept development. Concept Development in Nursing Foundations, Techniques, and Applications 129–159

Sheer B, Wong FKYM (2008) The development of advanced nursing practice globally. Journal of Nursing Scholarship 40(3):204–211

Stanley D, Stanley K (2018) Clinical leadership and nursing explored: a literature search. J Clin Nurs 27(9–10):1730–1743. https://doi.org/10.1111/jocn.14145. Epub 2018 Jan 11. PMID: 29076264

ten Hoeve Y, Jansen G, Roodbol P (2013) The nursing profession: public image, self-concept and professional identity. A discussion paper, pp 295–307

Thompson A (2019) An educational intervention to enhance nurse practitioner role transition in the first year of practice. Am Assoc Nurse Pract 31(1):24–32. https://doi.org/10.1097/jxx.0000000000000095

Throne S (2020) Rethinking Carper's personal knowledge for 21st century nursing. Nurs Philos 21:e12307. https://doi.org/10.1111/nup.12307

Tracy MF, O'Grady ET (eds.) (2019) Hamric and hanson's advanced practice nursing: an integrative approach, 6th ed. Elsevier. ISBN:978-0-323-44775-1

Treasurer B (2019) Develop these 3 types of courage in employees. https://hrdailyadvisor.blr.com/2019/06/25/develop-these-3-types-of-courage-in-employees/. Accessed 18 Dec 2021

Vaismoradi M, Salsali M, Ahmadi F (2011) Perspective of Iranian male nursing students regarding the role of nursing education in developing a professional-identity: a content analysis study. Jpn J Nurs Sci 8(2):174–183. https://doi.org/10.1111/j.1742-7924.2010.00172.x

Vinje HF, Mittelmark MB (2008) Community nurses who thrive: the critical role of job engagement in the face of adversity. J Nurses Staff Dev 24(5):195–202. https://doi.org/10.1097/01.NND.0000320695.16511.08. PMID: 18838896

Wald H (2015) Professional identity formation in medical education: reflection. Relationship, resilience. Acad Med 90(6):701–706. https://doi.org/10.1097/ACM.000000000000731

Walker LO, Avant KC (2011) Strategies for theory construction in nursing, 5th edn. Prentice Hall, Upper Saddle River, NJ

Walleck C (1991) Building a framework for dealing with ethical issues. AORN J 53(5):1248–1252

Woo BFY, Zhou W, Lim TW, Tam WWS (2019) Practice patterns and role perception of advanced practice nurses: a nationwide cross-sectional study. J Nurs Manag 2019(27):992–1004. https://doi.org/10.1111/jonm.12759

Wood LA, Olivier MA (2004) A self-efficacy approach to holistic student development. South Afr J Educ 24(4):289–294

APN Role Transition: Starting the Process

4

4.1 Introduction

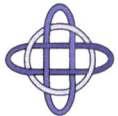

When a person gains a new skill or knowledge set, the person transitions to a higher level of critical and creative thinking incorporating the new skills/knowledge into their work. Role transition is a similar process where a person learns something new and incorporates the new skills/knowledge into a way of thinking and acting. This change has an identified process. Every person has gone through role transitions: student to work, child to adulthood, spouse to parent, or a professional transition from a staff position to a formal leadership role.

This book utilizes the Barnes (2015) NP role transition concept analysis to provide the framework of role transition. Although the research was on the nurse practitioner role, it can be applied to all APN roles (personal communication with H Barnes September 16, 2020). This chapter discusses the Barnes concept analysis that utilized the Walker and Avant's Wilson method to provide a process a person can follow to decrease stress and ambiguity that can surround role transitions. It is hoped that this chapter will spark your curiosity, give your creativity an outlet to build your skills/knowledge towards a successful role transition. Sometimes, just being aware that there is a similar process most people experience during role transition can provide hope and boost confidence.

© The Author(s), under exclusive license to Springer Nature Switzerland AG 2022
M. Kidner, *Successful Advanced Practice Nurse Role Transition*, Advanced Practice in Nursing, https://doi.org/10.1007/978-3-030-53002-0_4

Exemplar
Emily will be graduating soon as an advanced practice nurse. She has been hired as an APN for an outpatient primary care clinic. Emily previously worked as a generalist nurse on a surgical floor in the hospital. She is delighted to receive a job offer from this workplace facility because she completed two clinical rotations at the clinic as a student. Emily had two physicians as her clinical preceptors who encouraged her to work hard to understand clinically applied pathophysiology and increase her clinical skills. The physicians supported and guided Emily in her development of clinical decisions, diagnosis, and treatment plan development. Although she is transitioning from a generalist nurse to a primary care APN, she is feeling confident, has mentors in her new workplace, and has support from several other people and her family to start her new APN role.

4.2   Definitions

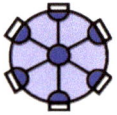

Antecedent   An antecedent is something that is required before an event, or activity and be completed. This preceding event, condition, or stimulus (the antecedent) will impact later developments of the desired outcome. For example, a nursing education is antecedent to practicing as a professional nurse. In this book, antecedent is used on context of a concept analysis. The antecedent is something that must happen, or be obtained, before the concept can occur (Walker and Avant 2011, p. 167).

Role transition   In the context of this book, role transition is specific to the process nurse's experiences when they increase their knowledge, skills, and critical thinking through graduate APN education with subsequent implementation of the APN role in clinical practice (Barnes 2015).

"Straddling"   *In the context of this book*, straddling refers to a specific time and process of role transition within the Barnes (2015) NP role transition concept analysis. Straddling refers to a time in which an APN student is a general nurse with the increasing knowledge and skills of the APN role, hence the student is effectively between two roles, or straddling two roles (a past and a future role) (Barnes 2015).

4.3   Role Transition

Role transition is unique and different for each person. Merriam-Webster dictionary (online accessed March 13, 2020) defines *"transition"* as a movement, development, or evolution from one form, stage, or style to another. As a nurse transitions from the role of a generalist nurse to an APN, there are many phases. Knowing there are similar emotions, barriers, facilitators, and processes can be helpful when you are feeling isolated or unsure of yourself during this APN role transition. The APN role is complex. Allow yourself to consider your thoughts, fears, eagerness, and excitement. These emotions will allow you to be creative in building your integrity and professional identity. The transitional process can be emotional and may seem difficult while you are immersed in your graduate education. Understanding the concept of role transition will help you be successful.

The expanded scope of practice of the APN requires the nurse to complete a graduate nursing education program including the mandatory clinical hours and testing to transition from generalist, or specialist nurse to APN. Yet, an APN is not just absorbing the knowledge base, but also integrating the core competencies of a different type of nursing with an expanded set of responsibility, authority, and accountability. Transitional times within nursing have been well studied and are identified with confusion, lower confidence, and personal disruption (Barnes 2015; Faraz 2019; MacLellan et al. 2015; Moran and Nairn 2018; Sangster-Gormley et al. 2013). Role transitions require time to adjust to the new role, responsibilities, and relationships (MacLellan et al. 2015).

4.3.1   Role Transition Concept Analysis

The Barnes' role transition concept analysis was a result of her research studying the transition of nurse practitioners through their graduate studies and into practice. This concept analysis is based on Walker and Avant's methodology (Walker and Avant 2011). Chapter 3 discussed concept analysis and methodology. The Walker and Avant methodology provides the research-specific steps to evaluate a concept, determine common themes, and provide specific case studies to clarify the concept. To keep the role transition discussion concise, only the essential concept analysis components will be explored. The three concept analysis components that are essential for APN students to understand the role transitional process are:

- Defining attributes
- Antecedents
- Consequences

4.3.2   Defining Attributes of the Barnes (2015) Role Transition Concept Analysis

A defining attribute is **an aspect** (a time or process) **that is highly characteristic of the concept** (Walker and Avant 2011). Barnes (2015) concept analysis of role transition describes four defining attributes of NP role transition: absorbing the new role; a shift from providing care to prescribing the care; straddling two identities; and mixed emotions. Let us examine each attribute:

1. **Absorption of the (new) role**—This is the time of high personal and professional development as one contemplates and moves from generalist nurse to APN. Absorption into the new role includes the engagement to gain technical skills, knowledge, and critical thinking through graduate-level education and clinical experiences. Emotions that are often expressed include: eagerness to learn, anticipation, fear of possible failure, and desire to become an APN (Barnes 2015).

2. **Shift from a nurse who provides care from a predetermined management plan to the nurse responsible to develop the complete plan**—This process starts with the recognition that the role of the APN is to provide healthcare through the advanced assessment, development, implementation, and evaluation of your own plans for patients. You will be assessing and developing healthcare management plans (in some countries this will include medication plans and diagnostic testing ordering and interpretation) for autonomous and collaborative clinical practices. The APN uses their advanced skills and competencies, increased clinical judgment, increased decision-making skills, and clinical leadership with authority in developing a patient's care. This shift combines the nature of the APN role with the understanding of the added responsibility of prescribing care (Barnes 2015).

   The recognition of this shift from generalist nursing to advanced practice nursing occurs through the development of your own comprehensive plans for your patients. The shift from *care provider to care prescriber* combines the generalist nurse knowledge with the new knowledge and skills of the APN education (Barnes 2015). Thus, you will be held accountable for your understanding of the role, decisions, and actions as you develop the plans which others (such as nurses, physical therapist, occupational therapist, respiratory therapists, or dieticians) may be part of the implementation.

   Although each person will react differently, a common thread of both excitement and worry are usually present during this part of role transition (Barnes 2015). There is wonder about developing highly successful plans and yet worry if your plans will be effective. This is an exciting time in your APN role development and learning about who you are—and will be—in this APN role.

A Note About Terminology

The Barnes role transition concept analysis uses **"a shift from providing care to prescribing the care."**

   In the context of this concept analysis "providing care" is the act of following another person's set of orders to implement the plan of care. Captured within "providing care" are all the aspects of nursing (such as critical thinking, autonomous decisions, case management, and patient education). This is a traditional role of generalist and specialist nurses.

   In the context of this concept analysis "prescribing care" is the act of developing the complete plan of care (all healthcare activities, referrals, outcome management, support, education, labs/tests, collaborations with other providers, and autonomous decisions pertaining to that patient and their support people) for a patient and may include the act of prescribing the medications in those countries where APNs have prescription privileges. Captured within this "prescribing care" is the unique APN clinical leadership with advocacy, understanding and use of evidence-based practice, collaboration, relationship building, and ethical decision-making. This is the critical role of APNs.

In some countries the terms to describe the person developing the plans of care and providing direct and indirect clinical care are: **"Healthcare Provider"** or in a primary care setting, a **"Primary Care Provider."** Healthcare providers include physicians, APNs, and other country-specific providers.

3. **Straddling two identities**—Many APN students will continue working as a nurse during their graduate education. As the level of education and clinical experiences increase, there is a time in which you are comfortable in your current nursing role yet see the potential of your upcoming role as APN. You will begin to understand how your new knowledge and skills impact your decisions. Gradually, there is a shift where you are looking more towards the APN role and less at your previous job/role (Barnes 2015).

Think of "straddling" as the process of stepping over a stream that is wider than a simple step but shorter than two steps. You will need to assess the stream, consider your option, plan your strategy to cross the stream without falling in the water. You will need to firmly set your foot, push off and reach out with determination to make the other side. The moment of pushing off is "straddling."

(a) **Mixed emotions**: Typically, the generalist nurse seeking to become an APN is already an expert in his or her field of nursing. APN students and new APNs often feel like an imposter or novice in the identity of the APN role (Thompson 2019). This sensation of being an APN imposter can occur when there is uncertainty in either didactic or clinical settings and can augment the feelings of straddling between the two identities: generalist nurse and APN. Chapter 7 expands the discussion of imposter syndrome. Conflicted feelings are a primary role transition attribute (Barnes 2015; Klein et al. 2020; Thompson 2019). The top emotions associated with role transition are:

- Excitement
- Stressed
- Anxious

- Nervous
- Overwhelmed
- Frustrated
- Feelings of inadequacy
- Ambivalence
- Uncertainty
- Not fitting in; not belonging; Isolation
- Longing to return to one's prior role
- Fear
- Eager anticipation
- Curiosity
- Anger
- Depersonalization
- Lack of personal accomplishment
- Imposter syndrome

(Barnes 2015; Klein et al. 2020; Thompson 2019)

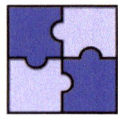

What other emotions could be possible?

_____
_____
_____

Circle all the emotions (from above) you are feeling now concerning your journey in becoming an APN. Know that these emotions are common and are part of the transition of a proficient or expert generalist nurse to the novice APN. Talking with fellow students, APNs, or friends can help you understand these emotions.

4.3.3   Questions on APN Role Transition Attributes to Guide Your Personal Journey

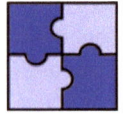

Review the four attributes of the Barnes NP role transition concept analysis (absorbed in new skills/knowledge, shift to prescriber of care, straddling two identities, and mixed emotions) and reflect on yourself and your personal journey. Answer the following questions.

Write down 1–2 learning activities/topic that excite you and make you want to be absorbed in the learning process of becoming an APN: _____

_____
_____

Can you think of some activities in your clinical work, or in your ability to develop plans where you find yourself moving towards a provider developing/prescribing the care versus providing care that someone else designed?_____

_____
_____
_____

In your current nursing role, what activities are you an expert?_____

_____
_____
_____
_____
_____

What activities will you be expected to do as an APN, but you are currently uncertain about, or are a novice?

_____
_____
_____
_____
_____
_____

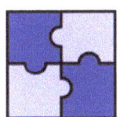

While you are obtaining your graduate education, you will straddle the roles as both a generalist or specialist nurse and an advanced practice nurse. Review the two tables of some recognized similarities and differences of the nursing roles of generalist, specialist, and advanced practice. Add your thoughts of other similarities or differences, then write or discuss with other students (or mentor) strategies to recognize the straddling, methods you can employ to help recognize and transition smoothly. Table 4.1 provides the similarities of all three nursing roles as all three roles use nursing theories and processes in critical thinking and providing care plus the differences in the complexity of thought and role responsibilities.

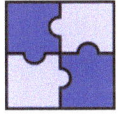

Table 4.1 Similarities and differences between generalist/specialist nurses and APN

Similarities within nursing roles

All three roles are advocates, mentors, and educators

All three roles teach patients, nurses, family, and community

All three roles complete assessments (although the APN assessments tend to be more detailed)

All three roles can work in collaboration and interprofessional teams

All three roles evaluate actions and patient responses to care provided, then make changes to improve care or outcomes

All three roles use nursing ethics and values

All three roles positively impact patients and communities by improving the quality of life of those under their care

Differences—APNs have increased knowledge and skills with enhanced accountability to:

Develop and monitor complex plans of care

Make autonomous *medical* diagnosis

Prescribe simple to complex medication management plans

When needed, the APN can refer patients to the appropriate provider for additional care

Order and interpret diagnostic tests and labs. Makes decisions based upon test results

Conduct complex skills based on education, clinical experience, location, and scope of practice

Generalist and specialist nurses follow plans of care developed by a healthcare provider (APN/physician) and use nursing diagnosis to guide care

Can you think of other similarities or differences?

Similarities	Differences

How do you think you will recognize when you are in the "straddling two roles" phase in your APN role transition? _____

_____

_____

What activities can you do to help you move from generalist nurse or specialist nurse to APN?

_____

_____

_____

How do you think you will know you have completed this phase of your role transition?

_____

_____

_____

_____

_____

4.3.4 Antecedents of the APN Role Transition Concept Analysis

Antecedents are events, or accomplishments, that must be achieved **before** the concept can be understood and personally incorporated (Walker and Avant 2011, p. 167). There are two types of antecedents in the Barnes (2015) role transition concept analysis: Personal and environmental.

4.3.5 Role Transition Personal Antecedents

Personal antecedents are activities that the person experiencing the role transition **must achieve** before the APN role transition can be successful. These antecedents are called "personal" because you have 100% control over the ability to achieve the activity. Chapter 5 has an in-depth discussion on personal antecedents as you use your developing APN professional identity during this time of APN role transition.

1. **Graduate-level education.** The requirement for the role of APN is a master's degree (ICN 2020) or a doctorate APN nursing degree (the graduate education must be specifically designed for the APN role). It is through formal graduate education that one learns knowledge and skills which add responsibility, accountability, authority, and autonomy to all APN nursing activities and ethics. The formal graduate education expands the nursing role and constitutes the APN role as distinctly different than a specialist nurse or generalist nurse (Barnes 2015). You have 100% control over the amount of effort and dedication you apply to be successful in your graduate-level education.
2. **Experience.** Obtaining proficient skills requires experiences to apply the knowledge and techniques of the skill. Experience is important for acquiring skill and developing competency (Benner 1983). Nursing and clinical experiences will impact your role transition by building confidence and skill proficiency (Barnes 2015). The required clinical practice hours of your APN education provide experiences to increase critical and creative thinking while developing clinical intuition as a provider over time. You have 100% control over the richness of your clinical experiences through your engagement and seeking of new experiences and patient complexities.
3. **Active disengagement from the previous role.** The APN student must disengage from the role of the generalist nurse in order to have openness to engage the new APN role (Barnes 2015). This is a necessary process, especially for nurses who continue to work as a generalist or specialist nurse while obtaining their graduate education. This disengagement process occurs when you eagerly look forward to the new possibilities you envision as an APN (Barnes 2015). The emotions associated with disengagement include curiosity, courage, anticipation, innovation, wonder, and seeking. You have 100% control over the timing in which you change your focus to your future as APN.
4. **Engagement.** When the APN student moves from a previous nursing role and becomes fully engaged in the future role of APN, engagement has occurred (Barnes 2015). Those who become actively engaged in the process of learning all aspects of the new role, seeking new information, actively preparing, and proactively modifying practice as knowledge and skills are gained will role transition

easier. You have 100% control to when you will be fully engaged in your education and new role as APN.

5. **Desire for feedback.** The student's desire for feedback from peers, colleagues, supervisors, and educators regarding the role performance is highly influential to role development (Barnes 2015; Jones 2014). Actively seeking feedback may increase sense of competence, self-efficacy, satisfaction and decrease role stress (Barnes 2015-2; Parschau et al. 2013). You have 100% control over requesting and how you receive feedback along with your response and embodiment of the feedback provided.

Learning a new set of knowledge or technical skills is improved when instructors, preceptors, or mentors provide honest and constructive feedback. Although, we all have some anxiety when being watched, most people still want constructive feedback on their progress. Plus, those students who receive feedback on their obtained knowledge will develop deeper knowledge, skills, and identity by incorporating the feedback to improve and grow while gaining competence, role clarity, and improved job performance (Al-Eraky et al. 2015; Algiraigri 2014; Lewis et al. 2019). If you feel uncertain about a process, knowledge, or decision, it is essential to seek guidance and feedback to help you recognize what you are doing well and areas where you need reinforced support to develop excellent habits.

Vulnerability is a risk when receiving positive or negative feedback. Actively seeking feedback shows the APN student is developing maturity, confidence, and professional identity. The emotions associated with receiving feedback range from fear, anxiety, and apprehension to curiosity and courage.

Steps for Receiving Feedback (Algiraigri 2014)
1. Do a self-assessment: Before receiving feedback, breakdown the skill/knowledge you completed into small steps and self-review each aspect.
2. Recognize the benefit from feedback: If no feedback is provided, ask for it. If feedback is provided, determine the actions you can make to improve.
3. Connection to your preceptor/professors: Work on developing trust and accountability to improve the quality of feedback.
4. Control your emotions: If the feedback provided is about the need to change or improve, expect an emotional response. Consider your emotional habits under stress and determine a plan to control your response.
5. Show appreciation: Tell people thank you for the feedback, explore details if needed, such as "how can I improve?" or "what can I expect if _____ complication arises?"

4.3.6 Questions to Review Personal Antecedents

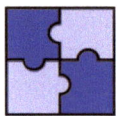

What aspects of disengagement do you recognize within yourself as you go through this process of moving away from your previous nursing role?

_____
_____

In what aspects of your future role as APN have you become engaged?

_____
_____

What experience have you had that you think has helped you in your education or role transition process?

_____
_____
_____
_____

Whom do you trust to provide you with feedback? _____
Why?_____
Are you currently receiving feedback concerning your APN education? Yes/No
If yes, describe a recent feedback session and how the process made you feel?

_____
_____
_____
_____
_____
_____

If no, identify 1–2 people whom you will ask for feedback during the next week?

_____
_____

How do you **feel** about your current ability to receive feedback?

_____
_____

You will receive negative feedback. Understanding how you respond is important in your role transition process. How do you handle negative feedback?

_____
_____
_____
_____
_____

4.3.7   Role Transition Environmental Antecedents

Environmental antecedents are activities, or processes, outside of the person's sole ability to obtain, yet must be accomplished before a successful role transition can occur (Barnes 2015). Although you cannot fully control the achievement of these antecedents, your response and participation will influence the outcomes of the environmental antecedents of job novelty, support, and formal orientation.

1. **Job Novelty**: Barnes describes *"job novelty"* has how similar or dissimilar the role is to the previous role which allows the individual *to use previous knowledge and skills* (Barnes 2015). A role with *low* job novelty offers fewer new challenges for the individual to gain new knowledge or skills. This occurs when you are an expert in the area of your course work thereby creating a situation where you may be less engaged with the new learning activities because of the similarities with your current role. An example can be a newborn nursery nurse returning to a graduate program for an APN neonatology degree.

   A role with *high* job novelty offers new skills and knowledge acquisition, and less opportunity to continue with previous skills. This occurs when the presented course is new to you and requires additional hours of reading and discussion to gain a true understanding of the content then have the ability to apply the knowledge to the clinical setting. An example can be an APN student learning to interpret abnormal 12 lead electrocardiograms (EKG) and respond with an evidence-based treatment plan to improve outcomes of patients with abnormal EKGs.

   Job novelty can also include responding to people, feedback, building relationships, and developing a personal leadership process in a new(novel) fashion. A graduate program provides the opportunity to try new responsibilities with enhanced accountability as you develop new plans of care. This time of graduate education provides you the opportunity to try new skills and leadership to improve your ability to lead and mentor others.

2. **Support:** A strong support network facilitates successful role transition and provide an important antecedent attribute (Barnes 2015; Jones 2014). The APN student must have support as an antecedent for a successful role transition (Barnes 2015). Support can come from other students, other APNs, faculties, instructors, workplace staff, physicians, friends, and family (or any of your stakeholders [see Chap. 2]). It is necessary to grow a support team to help during times of high frustration and to share in your celebrations of successes!

3. **Formal Orientation**: New graduates who complete a formal orientation or mentoring program into their new workplace may transition more easily, feel part of the team sooner, and have a higher sense of confidence and competence (Barnes 2015; Hernandez et al. 2017; Kowalski 2019). Many workplaces have formal orientation for the new APN. A formal orientation at your workplace may not have been developed yet. If you are unable to participate in a structured orientation, use your mentors and support people to help you transition into practice.

Do Not Underestimate Your Potential
If the APN role is new in your workplace and there is no formal orientation for APN, then after you complete your APN role transition you can help develop a formal orientation to help future APNs in your workplace!

Questions to Consider Your Environmental Antecedents

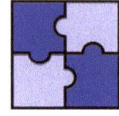

The higher the perceived novelty, the greater the personal dedication to development and learning. It is relevant to recognize that your APN education is building upon your nursing foundation, yet the APN role is vastly different, thus novel.

Compare your past nursing position to your anticipated APN practice. How similar are they?

_____

How do you feel your graduate education and clinical rotations are compared to your past nursing position considering job novelty? _____

If you are in a LOW novelty situation, what other aspects of your education can you focus upon where there is higher job novelty? _____

_____

What habits do you have now that you want to change when you enter a new and different nursing role? _____

_____

_____

List your support people and indicate if they are a mentor or preceptor:_____

_____

_____

_____

4.3.8 Consequences of Barnes (2015) Role Transition Concept Analysis

Consequences are the events that **result, or outcomes,** from occurrence of the concept (Walker and Avant 2011, p. 167). There are two consequences of this APN role transition: successful role transition and unsuccessful transition (Barnes 2015). Figure 4.1 provides a graphic representation of the APN role transition. In a successful APN role transition there is well-being, confidence, and competence in the role, with mastery of skills and autonomy of practice (Barnes 2015). Unsuccessful

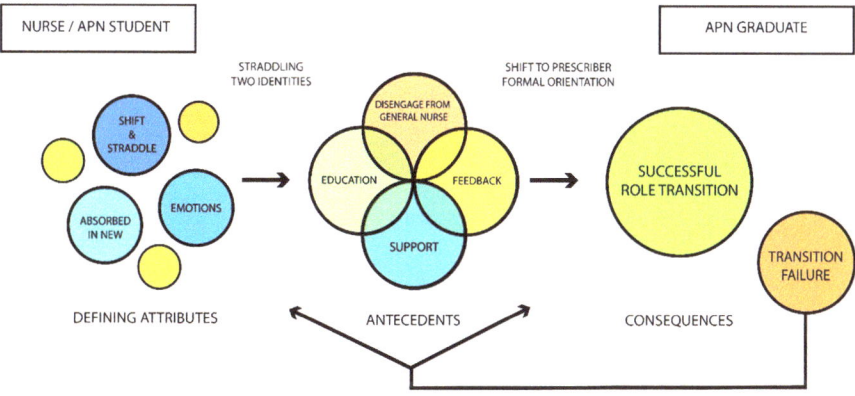

Fig. 4.1 APN role transition concept analysis. This figure is a new schematic based on Barnes (2015) role transition

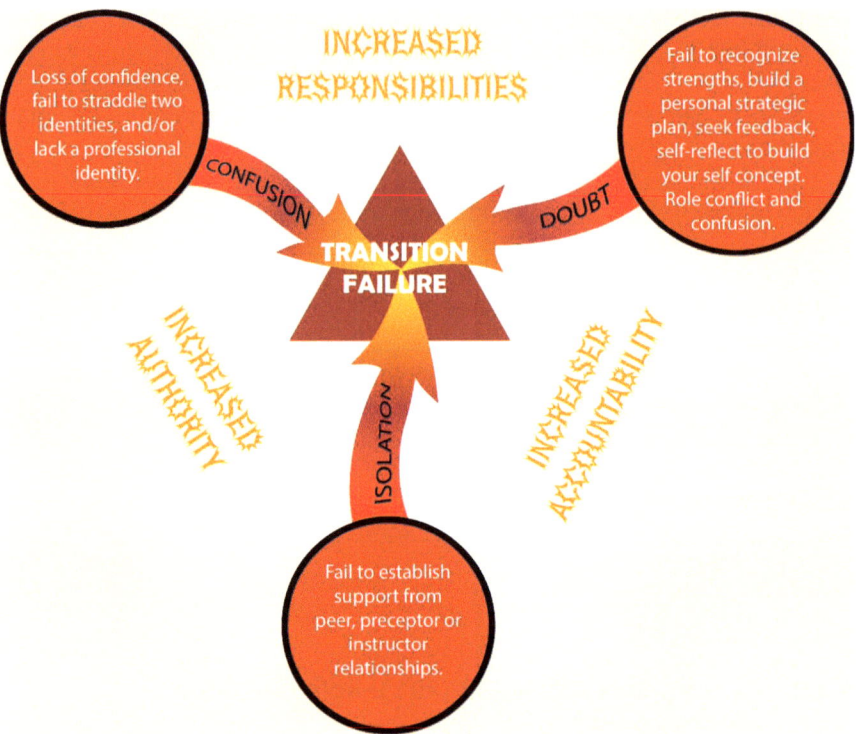

Fig. 4.2 Role transitional failure

APN role transition can result in resignation, turnover, or poor teamwork (Barnes 2015). Figure 4.2 is a graphic representation of APN role failure. In addition, unsuccessful role transition can include a loss of confidence, feelings of imposter syndrome, isolation, marginalization, and loss of identity (MacLellan et al. 2015).

Figure 4.2 is a graphic schematic of unsuccessful role transition created from the literature of Cruess (2006), Johnson et al. (2012), MacLellan et al. (2015), and Sun et al. (2016). Unsuccessful role transition can occur when the antecedents were not fully achieved. Loss of confidence, feelings of imposter syndrome, isolation, marginalization, loss of identity, turmoil, confusion, and/or self-doubt can result in transition failure and the person relinquishing APN practice (MacLellan 2015).

4.4   Role and Role Transition Stress

Emotion and role stress are entangled. Role stress can be a physical or psychological strain felt by a student when there is a perception of a lack of ability or resources for the student to perform the role (Sun et al. 2016). Role stress increases when the expectations of the experience are different than the actual experience and achievement. Role stress as an APN student can occur with:

- Incompatible role expectations
- Too much work is expected to be completed in too little time available
- Vague student role expectations without clear paths or support
- Assumptions of perfection being required
- Differences between the real-world application of theory with added ethical dilemmas
- Lack of coordination of patients, clinical instructors, and the educational program's expectations
- Lack of support from nursing, administration, peers, or physicians in clinical settings (Jones 2014; Reynolds and Mortimore 2021; Sun et al. 2016)
  Role stress as a new APN in practice can occur with:
- Uncertainty of actual role expectations in clinical practice
- Lack of clear role definition
- Role ambiguity and role incompatibility in the workplace
- Organizational culture that does not support APN
- Workplace passive aggression with vertical and lateral bullying/abuse
- Too much work is expected to be completed in too little time available
- Assumptions of perfection being required
- Differences between the real-world application of theory with added ethical dilemmas
- Lack of support from nursing, administration, peers, or physicians in clinical setting (Jones 2014; Reynolds and Mortimore 2021; Sun et al. 2016)

Negative responses to role stress during the APN graduate education is an indicator of future burnout and decreased engagement to either the educational process or to the final APN role (Sun et al. 2016). Professional identity is the strongest predictor within one's personal characteristics to respond in constructive ways to high role stress levels during academic education. As one develops a stronger professional identity, one gains more self-resiliency and lower role stress (Cruess 2006; Johnson et al. 2012; Sun et al. 2016).

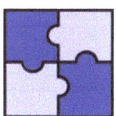

Review the concept analysis and determine where you are on each aspect: 0 means you have not started; 1 means you have not recognized the topic as a role transition process; 2 means you have recognized this process; 3 means you are actively working on it; and 4 means you have accomplished the process.

	0	1	2	3	4
Defining attributes					
I am absorbed in my education: I find all the work exciting	0	1	2	3	4
I am shifting from a provider of care to a prescriber of care	0	1	2	3	4

I feel like I am straddling two different identities as nurse and APN	0	1	2	3	4
I have mixed emotions: I am recognizing my emotions	0	1	2	3	4
Antecedents					
I am doing well in my graduate studies	0	1	2	3	4
I can sense my detachment as a generalist/specialist nurse	0	1	2	3	4
I feel like I am attaching to my new APN role and responsibilities	0	1	2	3	4
I want to know how I am doing in my progress of becoming an APN	0	1	2	3	4
I seek and obtain feedback well	0	1	2	3	4
Environment					
Job Novelty—I am eager/excited about my future as an APN	0	1	2	3	4
Support—I recognize I need support from friends and family	0	1	2	3	4
My current level of support from friends and family is _____	0	1	2	3	4
Support—I recognize the need of support from my peers/classmates	0	1	2	3	4
My current level of support from peers/classmates is _____	0	1	2	3	4
Support—I recognize I need support from my instructors	0	1	2	3	4
My current level of support from my instructors is _____	0	1	2	3	
Formal Orientation—Does the place you plan to work have one?	Yes	No	Do not know		
Consequences					
Success—I recognize my role transition is a formal process	0	1	2	3	4
My level of personal work and effort for a successful role transition	0	1	2	3	4

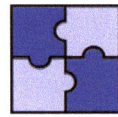

Now review your above answers and write at least three (3) steps you can take to ensure a successful role transition:

1. _____
   _____

2. _____
   _____

3. _____
   _____

4.5   Mentors

A review of the APN role transition and professional identity concept analyses reveal their model cases show the importance of finding mentors and support people to aid your successful transition. Many people have uncertainty concerning mentorship.

The word, "*mentor*" comes from the name of the friend Odysseus entrusted with the education of his son, Telemachus (in Greek mythology). Mentor was a wise and trusted man who would guide Telemachus from childhood into a man who became a great leader of his people. Today we seek "Mentors" in life as we seek to grow and understand life, our work, and our selves.

A Note: Molding your personal development is 100% your responsibility and 0% your mentor's responsibility. A mentor gives you a safe place to think, consider, and be creative in thought and action.

4.5.1 The Difference Between a Mentor and an Instructor/Preceptor

Mentoring is a process of providing inspiration, motivation, and guidance from a person with experience (the Mentor) to a person who is a novice (the Mentee) (Wensel 2006). It is based on a healthy and trusting relationship. Mentoring can be an important part of the development of self-image that impacts the growth and development of professional identity (Hernandez et al. 2017). In a mentor–mentee relationship, the mentee is encouraged to ask questions, seek guidance, discuss fears, excitement, problems, and successes. Mentoring is a one-on-one relationship. That relationship should include sponsorship, protection, challenges to consider and learn, and the sharing of advice (Kowalski 2019). Mentorship is not a graded student activity.

An Instructor/Preceptor is a formal educational role where the person has a formal relationship/contract to provide education, support, inspiration, and motivation for students. Almost always the instructor/preceptor will be required to supervise, evaluate, and grade the student's work. The establishment of a good learning environment where theory and practice complement each other, is dependent on the instructor and preceptor (Hong and Yoon 2021; Phuma-Ngaiyaye et al. 2017). Although the instructor(s) and preceptor(s) and student can develop a significant trust relationship, the instructor/preceptor's task is to complete the required knowledge and skills education in a clinical setting to improve clinical decision making with the translation of didactic knowledge into reality. After the completion of the graded course, an instructor or preceptor can then become a mentor because there is no evaluation or grade involved in the mentoring relationship.

4.5.2 The 5.5 Types of Mentors

As you go through your career you will seek advice and guidance from different people for different reasons. This section provides six different types of settings in which the mentor fills a specific need. Understanding the "5.5" types of mentors can help clarify in your mind that you are seeking a person to provide you with education, support, or motivation/inspiration.

0.5 = The "anti" mentor These are people with habits, reactions, or responses to situations that you do _not want to imitate_. You can learn from those actions in terms of what _not_ to do. However, you need to recognize the bad habits the "anti" mentor is using and make a conscious effort not to repeat the bad habits of that person (Stewart 2020). The mentorship (wisdom gained) from the "anti" mentor comes through the evaluation of the habit, reaction, or response that goes against your values or ideals. Developing a conscious process on how to avoid the disagreeable habit, reaction, or response is the learning and thus mentorship.

1 = The time machine mentor There are many great people who have walked this earth before us. We can learn so much by reading about those people and how they impacted others (their positive social influences). If you could have a conversation with anyone, who would it be? We now have technology to reach back and learn from so many great people from history's past. Some impressive nurses from the past include Florence Nightingale (1820–1910), Clara Barton (1821–1912), Maria Theresa of Austria (1717–1780), Hildegard Peplau (1909–1999), and Loretta Ford (1920–current). Today, you can easily access information about people of our past who shaped the future of nursing and life. The time machine mentor is the information found in books and the internet about past great people and events (Stewart 2020). Understanding how other nurses/people impacted patients, nurses and society can provide you with courage and inspiration. Building determination through the gained insight from people who have impacted (and still impact) society is mentorship.

2 = The micro mentor A micro mentor is the person we reach out and ask for their perspective. We can learn something from each person we meet, all we have to ask is, "what is your perspective on…" Then be a mindful listener. These mentors can give you insight into a lived experience (such as patients, family members, fellow students, instructors, and other stakeholders). Unexpected micro mentors are found simply by asking others to share their stories (Stewart 2020). It is through listening that creates the mentorship from a micro mentor. In nursing patients and colleagues are often micro mentors.

3 = The street mentor These are the people who know you very well! They stand beside you—in essence they walk down the street of life with you and support you such as your family and friends. Street mentors are people you have decided that can impact and direct your life. Typically, you do not have a formal mentor relationship with a street mentor, yet these people can have profound impacts on you. Some potential street mentors are your parents, grandparents, a sibling, or best friend. The mentorship is the inspiration, support, guidance, ability to share fears, joys, sorrows, and frustrations in a safe relationship allowing you to reflect on who you are and where you are going in life (Stewart 2020).

4 = The categorical mentor We know many people with a few great ideas, skills, or specific knowledge on a precise topic. A categorical mentor is a person from which you can learn a great knowledge, skills, or critical thinking (Stewart 2020). An example would be a person who can tracheal intubate patients in respiratory distress extremely well, and you would like to learn this skill. You would ask the person if they would train and supervise you to gain the ability to tracheal intubate as an expert. Categorical mentors usually have a hands-on skill, or a specific knowledge, or involve the ability to make complex critical decisions. This mentorship requires a short-term formal relationship of mentor–mentee.

5 = The worldview mentor The "traditional" mentor is the worldview mentor. This is the wise person with whom you want to develop a formal mentor relationship for a long-term commitment to obtain guidance, support, intense conversation, feedback, and a trusting relationship. This is the person you admire for their values, knowledge, skills, creative and critical thinking, ability in relationships, and their social influence/leadership style and impact (Stewart 2020). A worldview mentor would be the person to help guide you through APN novice to expert role transition.

> **Tips for the Mentee**
> - Develop a plan for yourself, your role, and your mentorships.
> - Know what type of mentor you need/want.
> - The most important aspect you will need as a successful mentee is your attitude!
> - You need to enter a mentorship with the desire to learn, ask questions, think, discuss, and share time and to be introspective about yourself with a wiliness to change.
> - Understand mentorship is not done to you but what occurs with you.

4.5.3 Finding a Mentor

"How do I find a mentor?" is a common question. The following six steps will guide you in collaborating with a mentor.

Step 1. Before looking for a mentor, be committed to the time and energy it takes to be a mentee. Below are additional aspects of consideration before committing to a mentor.

- The relationship is largely dependent upon you, your courage to reach out and ask for a mentorship and to maintain the relationship.
- Accept yourself where you are currently in your education and APN role transition.
- Believe that you and your profession are worth the effort.
- Imagine the possibilities; be curious.
- Be willing to consider multiple points of view.
- Be courageous to ask your mentor questions.
- Expect that a full mentorship is a long-term relationship.

Step 2. Review the people who have guided or impacted your life in the past. Once you understand who past mentors have been (what you admired in those people), you will be able to gain an insight into who will be able to help you become your best. Then determine who might become a mentor for you:

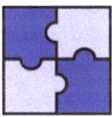

Who has inspired you to shift the direction of your life in a positive and constructive way? _____

Who provided or helped you to gain a deeper commitment to your personal values and ethical integrity?_____

Who provided you knowledge and guidance to gain a skill or technical competence?_____

Step 3. Determine what you are seeking to gain from your future mentor. This will clarify the type of mentor you are seeking. You can have more than one mentor at a time if you are methodical and plan well. Each takes time and effort from both people. Are you seeking …

- A technical skill or competency?
- Guidance and support during role transition?
- A specific area of knowledge or a skill?
- Personal growth, values, and ethic integrity?
- Understanding of the workplace culture?
- Other? _____

Step 4. Look at your workplace or graduate program for possible role models, support people, and mentors. Identify people who you will consider asking for a mentorship relationship. Write down your possible mentors in the categorical and worldview mentor types. If you have good internet access, your mentors can be anywhere in the world!

_____
_____
_____

Exemplar

When I was specializing in cardiology as an APN, my focus was on women. As I read more, I really enjoyed a certain author. I emailed her and asked if she would mentor me specifically in my growth on becoming an expert in female cardiovascular disease management. She agreed. I was not anyone special, but I had desire and determination to improve my skills and knowledge. We completed this relationship entirely via the internet and I am grateful for the opportunity. Have courage and reach out and ask!

Step 5. Have courage and simply ask that person(s).

- Most people are happy and willing to mentor others.
- If they are too busy, they will say so.
- When you ask, you can ask for a meeting to discuss how they would like to proceed in formal mentorship.
- Be specific in your request of mentorship: Is this for a worldview or categorical mentorship? Explain what you are seeking and that you are committed to the mentor relationship.

Step 6. Most commonly you will be asked about your goals. Read the section on a personal strategic plan and complete your personal plan before you ask someone to mentor you! Be prepared on your first visit with your mentor to clearly state what you are seeking.

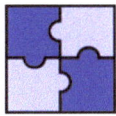

It is wonderful to have a person to ask questions, share fears, get feedback, and find support. For this assignment you need to find a person who will agree to be a categorical mentor: **a person to help you specifically through role transition and developing your professional identity**. This is a categorical mentorship because you are asking mentoring for a finite time frame (from the time you ask through your first year as an APN). Ideally, this should be an APN, however, it can be any person you want to gain their wisdom and guidance concerning role transition and/or professional identity formation. If you have reliable internet, this person can be anywhere in the world. This person may become a worldview mentor as your relationship grows.

1. Make a list of people you admire and why: Note: Admiring is not enough in terms of a mentor. Characteristics of a strong mentor are that they are experts in the field that you want to go into, they are patient, kind, yet capable of constructive criticism and they know how to communicate, they exhibit strong values that are similar to your values, and they are trustworthy.

   _____
   _____
   _____
   _____
   _____

2. You are looking for a wise person who can help your role transition and guide your self-reflection and professional identity formation.
Who will you ask? _____
3. When will you ask your potential mentor? _____

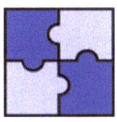

In groups of 3–5, or as an individual, brainstorm on ideas you feel will help you through your APN role transition mentorship.

What will help you have a successful role transition mentorship?

_____
_____
_____
_____
_____
_____

Ideas for successful role transition

1. Know that there is a process for role transition.
2. Recognize that your role transition will be emotional and hard work.
3. Acknowledge your emotions and frustrations.
4. Find support people to help you through your educational process and new role.
5. Learn about the new APN role, the impact of your culture, your government, and how society views nursing and APN.
6. Review the concept analysis and track your progress.
7. Use a journal (or this book) to record your progress and journey as you transition into an APN.
8. Develop positive coping skills.
9. Seek a mentor and establish a mentee–mentor relationship.

4.5.4   Other Supports

Psychologist Albert Bandura's life's work has been in human behavior and social cognitive theory. He developed the agentic theory in which the interplay of personal, behavioral, and environmental determinants become the product of human activity. People can affect their lives individually, by a proxy (society), or within a group. A group working towards a common cause that can share knowledge, skills, resources, and support can collectively help the group achieve the common purpose (Bandura 2018). Within your setting of your graduate program, developing friendships with fellow students to become a group with a common purpose (graduation and successful APN role transition) can become a strong support system to share and discuss experiences and dreams of the future. Many of these supportive relationships will become lifelong friendships.

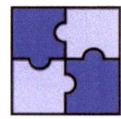

Review your student colleagues and identify two to five people whom you can set time to share your educational experiences, role transition process, and dreams of the future.

_____
_____
_____
_____

Set a date, time, and location for a student gathering and invite your student colleagues together.

4.6   Summary

This chapter provides a framework for increasing the understanding of the process of role transition through the use of the 2015 Barnes concept analysis on NP role transition. Although Barnes's research was exploring the nurse practitioner role transition, the process and concept can be applied to all APN students worldwide (personal communication with Hilary Barnes Sept. 16, 2020). The Walker and Avant's concept analysis methodology (2011) is utilized in providing discussion on the:

- Defining attributes
- Antecedents
- Consequences

The defining attributes are absorption into the new role; a shift from providing care prescribed by others to be the prescriber of care, straddling two identities; and mixed emotions.

The defining attribute of personal antecedents are identified activities that must be accomplished for a successful role transition and include: the completion of a graduate education in APN nursing; disengagement from the previous generalist/specialist nursing role; and engagement to the new APN role. The importance of instructors, preceptors, and mentors cannot be understated to achievement of the antecedents.

The defining attribute of environmental antecedents required for a successful APN role transition includes: a high job novelty; support (mentors, preceptors, instructors, and others); and a formal orientation at the APN workplace after graduation.

The consequences of role transition are a successful or unsuccessful APN role transition from a generalist nurse to APN and role transition from a graduate program to successful transition into the APN role (see Chap. 7).

References

Al-Eraky MM, Donker J, Wajid G, Van Merrienboer JJ (2015) Faculty development for learning and teaching of medical professionalism. Med Teach 37(4 Suppl 1):S40–S46. https://doi.org/1 0.3109/0142159x.2015.1006604

Algiraigri AH (2014) Ten tips for receiving feedback effectively in clinical practice. Med Educ Online 19(1):25141. https://doi.org/10.3402/meo.v19.25141

Bandura A (2018) Toward a psychology of human agency: pathways and reflections. Perspect Psychol Sci 13(2):130–136. https://doi.org/10.1177/1745691617699280

Barnes H (2015) Nurse practitioner role transition: a concept analysis. Nurs Forum 50(3):137–146

Barnes H (2015) Exploring the factors that influence nurse practitioner role transition. J Nurse Pract 11(2):178–183. https://doi.org/10.1016/j.nurpra.2014.11.004

Benner P (1983) Uncovering the knowledge embedded in clinical practice. Image J Nurs Sch 15(2):36–41

Cruess RL (2006) Teaching professionalism. Clin Orthop Relat Res 2006(449):177–185. https://doi.org/10.1097/01.blo.0000229274.28452.cb

Faraz A (2019) Facilitators and barriers to the novice nurse practitioner workforce transition in primary care. J Am Assoc Nurse Pract 31:6;364–370. https://doi.org/10.1097/JXX.0000000000000158

Hernandez PR, Bloodhart B, Barnes RT, Adam AS, Clinton SM, Pollack I et al (2017) Promoting professional identity, motivation, and persistence: benefits of an informal mentoring program for female undergraduate students. PLoS One 12(11):e0187531. https://doi.org/10.1371/journal.pone.0187531

Hong KJ, Yoon HJ (2021) Effect of nurses' preceptorship experience in educating new graduate nurses and preceptor training courses on clinical teaching behavior. Int J Environ Res Public Health 18(3):975. https://doi.org/10.3390/ijerph18030975. PMID: 33499327; PMCID: PMC7908293

International Council of Nursing (2020) Guidelines on advanced practice nursing 2020. Geneva. https://wwwicnch/system/files/documents/2020-04/ICN_APN%20Report_EN_WEBpdf. Accessed 17 Apr 2020

Johnson M, Cowin LS, Wilson I, Young H (2012) Professional identity and nursing: contemporary theoretical developments and future research challenges. Int Nurs Rev 59(11):562–569. https://doi.org/10.1111/j.1466-7657.2012.01013.x

Jones ML (2014) Role development and effective practice in specialist and advanced practice roles in acute hospital settings: systematic review and meta-synthesis. J Adv Nurs 49(2):191–209

Klein CJ, Lizer S, Cooling M, Pierce L (2020) Advanced practice provider perspectives on organizational strategies for work stress reduction. West J Nurs Res 42(9):708–717. https://doi.org/10.1177/0193945919896606

Kowalski K (2019) Mentoring. J Contin Educ Nurs 50(12):540–541. https://doi.org/10.3928/00220124-20191115-04

Lewis et al (2019) A focus on feedback: improving learner engagement and faculty delivery of feedback in hospital medicine. Pediatr Clin N Am 66:867–880. https://doi.org/10.1016/j.pcl.2019.03.011

MacLellan L, Levett-Jones T, Higgins I (2015) Nurse practitioner role transition: a concept analysis. J Am Assoc Nurse Pract 27(7):389–397. https://doi.org/10.1002/2327-6924.12165. Epub 2014 Sep 4

Moran GM, Nairn S (2018) How does role transition affect the experience of trainee advanced clinical practitioners: qualitative evidence synthesis. J Adv Nurs 74:251–262. https://doi.org/10.1111/jan.13446

Parschau L et al (2013) Positive experience, self-efficacy, and action control predict physical activity changes: a moderate mediation analysis. Br J Health Psychol 18:395–406. https://doi.org/10.1111/j.2044-8287.2012.02099.x

Phuma-Ngaiyaye E, Bvumbwe T, Chipeta MC (2017) Using preceptors to improve nursing students' clinical learning outcomes: a Malawian students' perspective. Int J Nurs Sci 4(2):164–168. https://doi.org/10.1016/j.ijnss.2017.03.001. PMID: 31406737; PMCID: PMC6626121

Reynolds J, Mortimore G (2021) Transitioning to an ACP: a challenging journey with tribulations and rewards. Br J Nurs 30(3):166

Sangster-Gormley E, Frisch, Schreiber R (2013) Articulating new outcomes of nurse practitioner practice. J Am Assoc Nurse Pract 25;12:653–658. https://doi.org/10.1002/2327-6924.12040

Stewart D (2020) Mentorship. Conference presentation at fellows of the American Association of Nurse Practitioners Winter Meeting, 2020 Feb. 29; Austin, Texas

Sun L et al (2016) The impact of professional identity on role stress in nursing students: a cross-sectional study. Int J Nurs Stud 63:1–8. https://doi.org/10.1016/j.ijnurstu.2016.08.010

Thompson A (2019) An educational intervention to enhance nurse practitioner role transition in the first year of practice. Am Assoc Nurse Pract 31(1):24–32. https://doi.org/10.1097/jxx.0000000000000095

Walker LO, Avant KC (2011) Strategies for theory construction in nursing, 5th edn. Prentice Hall, Upper Saddle River, NJ

Wensel TM (2006) Mentor or preceptor: what is the difference? Am J Health Syst Pharm 63(17):597. https://doi.org/10.2146/ajhp060121

Finding Paths to Successful Transitions

5

5.1   Introduction

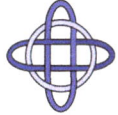

Formation of a nurse's professional identity starts with the first thoughts of wanting to be a nurse (Pullen 2021). Your image of "nurse" has changed with your education and your clinical practice as a generalist nurse, and development of your expertise through your nursing experiences. Your identity as APN began when your curiosity of the APN role started. You are now in the process of role transition from a generalist nurse to APN.

Reflection of your deep, personal, internalized process of who you are as APN is your professional image which is the foundation of your professional identity (Pullen 2021). Understanding and learning how to develop a professional identity is as essential to your success as an APN as the technical knowledge and skills you need to provide excellent healthcare to your future patients (Cruess 2006; Nocerino et al. 2020). Your identity as an APN will guide your ethical integrity and support your self-concept and confidence in your knowledge, skills, and abilities to help others. This chapter provides you with an in-depth understanding of the complexities and relevance of the development of your APN professional identity.

© The Author(s), under exclusive license to Springer Nature Switzerland AG 2022
M. Kidner, *Successful Advanced Practice Nurse Role Transition*, Advanced
Practice in Nursing, https://doi.org/10.1007/978-3-030-53002-0_5

Exemplar

John is in his last year in his APN education. He recently started a new pediatric clinical rotation in a hospital he has never worked. His first week was difficult as he felt the nursing staff was unfriendly towards him. He found himself wondering why the nurses were unfriendly to him as this new APN could bring a new level of education to the profession. John felt nursing was a profession designed to bring improved health to patients and communities. The following day, John found several of the nurses talking and pointing at him. He went to visit with the staff and quickly realized that this nursing staff had never been introduced to the APN role and they felt he had overstepped his nursing role and was "playing doctor." John explained the similarities and differences between a general nurse and an APN. He explained that although he was an expert in surgical nursing, he was learning a new role and needed their understanding and support as nurse and APN. John made a path to a successful pediatric clinical rotation and developed true friends and support from those nurses.

5.2   Definitions

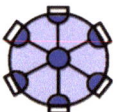

Profession A *profession* is a paid occupation requiring specialized knowledge and often long and intensive academic preparation whose core element is work based on the mastery of that complex body of knowledge and skills (https://www.merriam-webster.com/dictionary/profession 2020). A healthcare professional is:

- Governed by a code of ethics
- Committed to competency
- Focused on the promotion of the public good
- Pledged to integrity, morality, and altruism
- Accountable to those they serve and to society (Cruess 2006)

Professionalism *Professionalism* is the conduct, aims, or qualities that characterize or mark a profession or a professional person. Professionalism is the resulting behavior of the profession's socialization process of formal education where students develop personal and professional values and the culture of the profession (values, attitudes, and specialized skills and knowledge) (Cruess 2006; https://www.merriam-webster.com/dictionary/professionalism).

Professional identity *Professional identity* is one's conduct, aims, belief systems, and qualities that characterize a profession in which the person belongs. The person is committed to incorporation into self the values, practices, and purpose inherent in the role and profession in which one is a constituent (Johnson et al. 2012; https://www.merriam-webster.com/dictionary/professionalism).

APN Professional identity The *APN professional identity* is the inclusive personal paradigm of what it means to be an APN through embodiment of the rules, beliefs, and practice activities (Anderson et al. 2020). This paradigm includes:

- The values and beliefs held by APNs that guide thinking, actions, and interactions
- The commonly held APN attributes
- An understanding of how the APN profession compares and differentiates themselves from another professional groups
- A personal understanding and incorporation of self-values
- Commitment to the purpose inherent in the APN role (to provide high-quality healthcare)
- Advanced APN nursing knowledge, skills, and decision-making (Anderson et al. 2020; Sun et al. 2016; ten Hoeve et al. 2014)

Your professional identity provides a framework for you to organize your knowledge and apply your values and ethics that guide and drive your behavior (Johnson et al. 2012).

Self-concept *Self-concept* is the mental image one has of oneself including the personal understanding of perceived attributes. Your self-concept includes your personal values, behaviors, beliefs, assumptions, and attitudes. These become the contextual influences that inform your ethical decision-making process (Barlow et al. 2018; Walleck 1991). It is the inner knowledge of yourself and the way you think about yourself (Johnson et al. 2012; ten Hoeve et al. 2014). Self-concept is tied to professional identity yet is distinct (Johnson et al. 2012; ten Hoeve et al. 2014).

5.3   Understanding Professional Identity Formation

Novice APN role transition has been described as both stressful and turbulent, marked by the shift from an experienced, expert status in the generalist nurse role to an inexperienced novice in the APN role (Barnes et al. 2021; Gutierrez and Morais 2017; Pullen 2021). This role transition can impact one's professional identity and often leads to a temporary decreased confidence and job satisfaction which can impair role development (Barnes et al. 2021). However, gaining knowledge on professional identity changes through APN role transition can improve your self-efficacy, confidence, and role transition. Spending time in introspection and discussion can greatly enhance your self-concept and professional identity as APN.

Professional identity as "nurse" develops when a nurse reflects and internalizes the core values, norms, characteristics, and scope of practice of the nursing profession (Ageiz et al. 2021). As you engage in continued personal and professional development while gaining experiences in the clinical setting, your professional identity gains a stronger commitment to APN nursing. Subsequently, as you role transition from general nurse to APN, your professional identity evolves with the integration of critical/creative thinking and clinical reasoning using the core values as you begin to think, feel, and perform as an APN (Pullen 2021).

Your professional identity is nurtured, and changed by engaging with other APNs, being mentored, working with interprofessional team members, and increasing your knowledge. Professional identity is strengthened through a commitment to lifelong learning, service to the community, achievement of advanced degrees and certifications with sharing of that knowledge, and membership in APN professional organizations (Ageiz et al. 2021; Pullen 2021).

APN professional identity formation is complex and often occurs through a subconscious development of the understanding of self as an APN. However, an APN can deeply enrich their professional identity through understanding different aspects of identity and processes that can aid the formation of a strong and positive APN professional identity. A fundamental goal of professional identity formation is the development of professional attitudes and behaviors with a deeply internalized ethical and moral duty to safe, effective, quality, and autonomous patient care that will guide how APNs conduct themselves in their day-to-day practice (Ageiz et al. 2021; Kline et al. 2020). The personal formation of the understanding of who we are and who we are to become is a combination of socialization and personal psychological review (Kline et al. 2020). The socialization aspects include:

- The influence of experienced professional role models
- Immersion in a community of practice
- Clinical encounters with patients
- The code of nursing ethics in your country
- The scope of APN practice in your country
- Support of the role from key stakeholders

You can be proactive in the development of your professional identity by utilizing a structured process with forethought and preplanned actions. The activities APN students can accomplish during their graduate education to consciously develop their personal professional identity to the APN role can include:

- Build trust relationships: Be kind, spend time with others, and actively listen to promote relationship building.
- Work on group projects and be an active participant on those projects.
- Develop and implement patient education activities.
- Set a time to be introspective and look at your professional identity formation (such as completing the activities in this book).

- Discuss professional identity and role transition with your peers, preceptors, mentors, and instructors.
- Review, discuss, and internalize the ethical and moral duty to provide safe and high-quality patient care.
- Engage in clinical discussions with other APN students and APNs.
- Increase your APN knowledge (Barlow et al. 2018; Gutierrez and Morais 2017; Karanikola et al. 2018; Pullen 2021; Wald 2015; Walleck 1991).

As an APN clinician:

- Seek and take leadership roles (formal and informal)
- Be active in evidence-based practice and research
- Participate in quality improvement projects
- Use informatics
- Exemplify patient-centered care through your actions and healthcare plans
- Promote patient safety
- Maintain cultural sensitivity
- Use effective communication and collaboration
- Advocate for equal resource utilization
- Support environmental health of all staff and patients
- Be active in nursing and healthcare organizations
- Project your APN image in all you do
- Continue your education and certificates on activities you want to pursue
- Participate in committee or community activities
- Embrace diversity, equity, and inclusion
- Provide a professional presentation
- Teach a course
- Be a mentor
- Engage in academic and clinical discussions with nurses, APNs, and other healthcare professionals (Barlow et al. 2018; Gutierrez and Morais 2017; Karanikola et al. 2018; Wald 2015; Walleck 1991).

5.4   Understanding Yourself Now

The development of your professional identity does not occur in a straight line. There will be gains and there will be setbacks as you view and review your personal growth, self-accountability, self-resiliency, and confidence as you progress through your education towards an APN role (Cruess et al. 2019). Your personal habits and beliefs will impact your professional identity. The identity of an APN includes the set of knowledge and practices that APNs do worldwide. Your professional identity includes the sharing of global values and ethics as an APN that you identify as a person and nurse (Gutierrez and Morais 2017). As you progress through your education and clinical experiences, you will develop a sense of competence and confidence that is critical for the stabilization of your personal identity. This is the foundation of your professional identity formation.

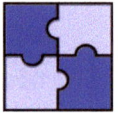

Before you can determine how your professional identity will change in the APN role, it is important to understand who you are before you proceed to develop, or refine, your APN professional identity. Answering the following questions will help guide your thoughts on who you are now and who you are becoming. As you move from the generalist role to the APN role ("*straddle*" in the Barnes concept analysis) you will be both looking back at yourself as nurse and forward at your future as APN. Please answer these questions. There are no wrong answers!

What does "Professional identity" mean to you at this moment?

_____
_____
_____

How do you think a person can gain personal and professional identity?

_____
_____
_____
_____

How do you think role transition can impact professional identity?

_____
_____
_____
_____
_____

Your outward reflection of your deep, personal, internalized process of who you are as APN is your professional image which is the foundation of your professional identity (Pullen 2021). As previously discussed, introspection is a needed skill in a structured and planned process of professional identity formation. Introspection is a great source of personal knowledge and allows:

- Knowledge that is not possible in any other way
- Revelation of connections between different experiences and responses
- The cause and meaning of previous activities and accomplishments to be understood
- The linking of a social or professional group to self for professional identity attachment

- A review of personal pursuits, goals, and progress (Bandura 2018; Cherry 2020; Pullen 2021)

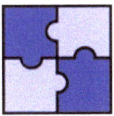

Following are some personal questions to consider aiding in your introspection.

What is your personal philosophy of nursing that is your foundation of your practice?

For me, nursing is _____

_____

_____

_____

From a general perspective, how do you describe your beliefs about the APN roles?

I believe that APN is _____

_____

_____

What are your beliefs about providing care to patients?

_____

_____

_____

_____

What is your personal belief on what is health?

I believe "health" is _____

_____

_____

_____

The environment?

I believe the environment _____

_____

_____

_____

How do caring relationships promote health, healing, and effective communication and collaboration?

_____

_____

_____

_____

How does patient-centered care ensure safe, quality patient care and promote the achievement of positive patient outcomes? _____

_____

_____

_____

_____

Review your clinical experience and write about a time when a patient allowed you to demonstrate your personal values (personal values will be discussed in Chap. 6).

_____

_____

_____

_____

_____

- As you review your answers, you should be able to recognize that you are building your own understanding of nursing, the APN role and its possibilities, your perceptions of care and what values you base your care and decisions upon. These thoughts are the core concepts of your professional identity. In addition, your professional identity is impacted by those around you along with the environment in which you practice. It is meaningful for you to review the above questions now, when you graduate, and after you graduate in order to recognize the influences on your professional identity and make your personal choice in what you believe and how those beliefs direct your care and your understanding of the APN role.

5.4.1 Personal Factors of Your Role Transition That Guide Your Professional Identity

Personal factors of your professional identity that develop through your APN role transition are factors that you have control over and can choose to achieve or ignore. Chapter 4 provided an in-depth discussion of the concept analysis of role transition by Barnes (2015). As you are now aware, the development of your professional identity as APN is changing, contextual, uniquely personal and you have personal control over many aspects of what you choose to incorporate in your paradigm of what is an APN and how you fit within your paradigm. There are personal factors that impact the development of your professional identity as an APN. These include:

- Your perceived traditions of current workplace policy (such as caring for the poor in the emergency room or pediatric pain management).
- Your skills and proficiency of those skills (your current technical skill/abilities to achieve the task in question).
- Your advanced knowledge and ability to apply that knowledge in clinical settings.

- Your level of confidence in deviating from workplace norms and culture when you know you are correct.
- Your past experiences as a nurse in providing care.
- Your past experiences in relationship to how you were respected by peers, staff, and physicians (this determines the level of trust and integrity others have placed upon you).
- Your perceived social norms of the workplace and nursing (your courage, self-confidence, and self-resiliency to be an advocate when faced with a dilemma).
- Your ability to share and talk after significant events.
- Your personal value system, beliefs, and assumptions that guide your personal moral code and ethics.
- Your sense of belonging to a group of people (APNs).
- Your desires for the future (will you be an advocate for others?) (Barlow et al. 2018; Gutierrez and Morais 2017; Karanikola et al. 2018; Nocerino et al. 2020; ten Hoeve et al. 2014; Wald 2015; Walleck 1991).

These contributing personal factors of the development of your professional identity centers on the recognition of personal perceptions, knowledge, values, and behaviors. The importance of personally reviewing self-concept and the professional identity process is to provide you with a guide and cornerstone during times of moral or ethical conflicts that are inevitable in the healthcare professions. You will be responsible for life and death decisions, and the consequences of the skills/knowledge used for your decisions (Wald 2015). This self-awareness will impact how you interact with patients and ultimately impact the quality of provided patient care (Barlow et al. 2018; Karanikola et al. 2018).

The specific APN role transition personal factors of the Barnes role transition concept analysis (Barnes 2015) can then be added to the context of professional identity awareness. The concept analysis lists four personal factors to acquire for a successful transition to the APN role. They are:

- Graduate education
- Clinical experiences
- Focusing on the future
- Desire for feedback

5.4.2 Graduate Education

This dedicated graduate-level education sets the APN role apart from generalist nursing with exclusive advanced nursing knowledge, skills, and critical thinking applied to clinical practice for APNs to provide high-quality, effective, and safe clinical and preventative healthcare. Your professional identity concerning your academic knowledge is changing with your graduate education as you embrace the core nursing values through a new paradigm as autonomous healthcare provider. Graduate education is an immersion in knowledge, engagement with student peers, faculty, preceptors, and patients providing a context to develop personal concepts and processes on integrating critical thinking and clinical reasoning to become an APN in thought and action (Pullen 2021). You will continue to develop your identity as an APN through your lifelong learning.

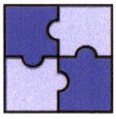

List at least three topics of knowledge that you have learned that is specific to the APN role and will impact how you provide healthcare in the future and explain why those topics are important to you:

_____
_____
_____
_____
_____
_____
_____

- APN education is dynamic and encompasses both the formal graduate-level education and the education received at the workplace after graduation. Personal factors to maximize this combined formal and workplace education requirement include self-efficacy and the presence of achievement goals (Grosemans et al. 2020). Both self-efficacy and stated goals relate to how you understand yourself and evaluate your perception of your APN competencies. Subsequently, your self-efficacy and stated academic achievement goals have been found to predict performance and the capacity of learning new competence. Yet, these personal factors are also dynamic and will change throughout your APN role transition process. It is anticipated that as you gain knowledge, skills, critical and creative decision-making with the ability to apply these in your clinical setting, you will gain confidence and higher self-efficacy. Likewise, your achievement goals will change as you continually meet your stated goals.

- Many APN students were experts in their original fields of practice with concurrent high self-efficacy. The abrupt change to novice APN status can be challenging and often underestimated (Reynolds and Mortimore 2021) which can impact self-efficacy.
- Learning to set academic achievement goals during graduate education can led to the habit of setting and monitoring achievement goals that translate to an easier transition into clinical practice (Grosemans et al. 2020).

5.4.3   Clinical Experience as an Autonomous Healthcare Provider

Your clinical activities as an APN student provide you with time, patients, and context to translate theory into practice through your experience as an autonomous clinical provider. How you feel about yourself as an APN is directly related to your clinical experiences. Your feelings towards your personal capabilities will change as you continue through your education and throughout your career as you experience the role and consequences (positive or negative) of your clinical decisions as you develop from a novice APN to an expert APN. A significant part of professional identity is the embodiment of professional attitudes and behaviors embedded in your ethics that guide how you conduct yourself as an APN (Ageiz et al. 2021; Kline et al. 2020). Thus, the socialization and contextual framework of your professional identity is obtained through your clinical rotations, your experiences, and the discussions about your experiences with student peers, faculty, preceptors, close support people, and other experienced professional role models.

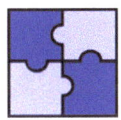

List at least three people who you are comfortable with in discussing your clinical experiences and who will help you gain an understanding of yourself through these experiences:

_____

_____

_____

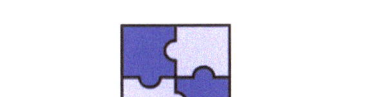

In your opinion, how should an APN present themselves (act) during clinical practice? Why do you think that?

_____

_____

_____

_____

_____

5.4.4   Focus on the Future: Active Disengagement from Your Previous Nursing Role

Active disengagement from your previous nursing role encourages you to be curious and seek new knowledge allowing engagement to the new APN role, the identity as APN, and the possibilities the future holds as APN. Each of us have made a life transition: adolescent to adulthood, University to our first nursing job, perhaps even different positions within your generalist nursing role. Each transition requires you to go from a place of personal comfort to a feeling of insecurity. Yet, when you completed that transition, you successfully left the security of your past position and embraced the future. It is not different as you transition from a generalist nurse to an APN. You will need to let your generalist nursing activities and processes remain in the past. You will need to embrace the future as an autonomous healthcare provider. Disengagement does not mean you forget your nursing foundation. The APN role is built upon your past nursing knowledge, skills, and experiences. Yet, the APN role is different than the generalist nursing role as an APN is responsible for many of the clinical decisions and plans for the patient's care which requires a different set of critical and creative thinking, an enhanced level of clinical leadership, and a unique set of nursing knowledge to reach the high level of accountability and responsibility of the APN role.

Some students must continue to work during their APN education. If you are working as a nurse during your education, then it is necessary for you take time and be introspective with forethought about where you were in your past (current) role, what you are currently learning about the APN role, and where you see yourself in future (Barnes 2015). It is common to feel that you may be abandoning your coworkers as you go through your graduate education (Bleich 2017). In addition, graduate education is often filled with unknown expectations, complexities and challenges which can compound feelings of emotional uncertainty and a desire to remain in the comfort of the past through a persistent attachment to your last nursing role. For your successful role transition, development of a healthy self-concept and professional identity, you need to embrace your education and eagerly anticipate the APN role as a unique and different nursing role.

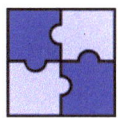

On a scale of 0–10 with "10" being completely ready to let your general nursing role remain in your past as a foundational stone to your APN role, determine where you are today:

0   1   2   3   4   5   6   7   8   9   10

Why did you choose that number of readiness and what might it mean to your role transition process?

_____
_____
_____
_____
_____

- If you have chosen "0" or "1" then please reach out to a trusted faculty member and discuss your current difficulties with disengagement from your last (or current) nursing job and the potential impact you may have as you progress.
- Continuing to work during your education can create wonderful opportunities for you to apply what you are learning to your daily practice. Yet, staying entrenched into general nursing process can create additional barriers in your role transition. The crucial understanding is the recognition that there is a past and future to your nursing and they are different.

5.4.5   Focus on the Future: Engagement in the New APN Role, the Identity as an APN, and the Possibilities the Future Holds as an APN

The shift from generalist nursing to an APN role requires disengagement from the generalist nursing role with the curiosity and desire to be engaged in a new way of applying nursing principles and processes in an autonomous healthcare provider paradigm. As a student, this engagement includes your hopes, dreams, and curiosity of the future as APN. Engagement of the nursing role can be filled with both eager anticipation and worry of the future. Transitions, the embodiment of a positive professional image, gaining the knowledge and skills, and the development of a positive self-concept can be challenging. Yet, as you go through a structured process of review and development of your professional identity you will find your inner strengths to help you obtain a success transition to the APN role.

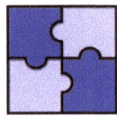

On a scale of 0–10 with "10" being completely ready to engage and embrace the APN role and your transitional process of becoming an APN.

0   1   2   3   4   5   6   7   8   9   10

Why did you choose that number of readiness and what might it mean to your role transition process?

_____
_____
_____
_____

5.4.6   Desire for Feedback to Help Personal Understanding of Current Development and Creation of Curiosity for the Future

Having a desire to seek and receive feedback to help guide your development process is the first step in translating didactic education into clinical wisdom. One of the personal challenges through your lifelong learning is developing a personal understanding that you have truly been able to understand and apply a topic or skill proficiently. One of the best ways to gain an understanding of how well you have progressed is the ability to ask for feedback. In the Barnes (2015) role transition model, Dr. Barnes used "desire for feedback." One must have enough confidence and positive self-concept to desire feedback. The desire means you will seek honest feedback from experienced clinicians that can provide feedback that will guide and inspire you to even greater knowledge and skills. Obtaining both the desire and the ability to receive feedback is imperative in development of a strong clinical foundation for clinical decisions (Barnes 2015; Farčić et al. 2020).

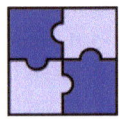

Explain how you think receiving feedback will impact your professional identity:

_____
_____
_____
_____
_____

5.5   Environmental Factors to Role Transition and Professional Identity Formation

Environmental factors are those which you do not have direct control over yet will impact either the process or your professional identity formation. All human activities and outcomes are the products of social influences, and the behaviors individuals engage within a set of environment factors (Bandura 2018). Therefore, you have the ability to impact events and the course of actions your life can take (Bandura 2018). The ability to have forethought allows you to realize your desired future; self-reactiveness allows you to adapt behavior standards to compare your performances; and self-reflectiveness allows you to review your challenges in the setting of meaning and ethics (Bandura 2018). These activities are directly connected to the process of professional identity enhancing your role transition and help you gain your APN professional identity.

There are four major environmental factors identified in APN role transition literature:

1. **Support** (Barnes 2015; Wensel 2006; Herdanez et al. 2017; Kowalski 2019; Smith et al. 2019; ten Hoeve et al. 2014)
2. **Socialization** on context of the learning experiences and laws/regulations impacting nursing (Kline et al. 2020; ten Hoeve et al. 2014; Bandura 2018; Barlow et al. 2018; Karanikola et al. 2018; Walleck 1991)
3. **A post-graduate transitional orientation** (Barnes 2015; Barnes et al. 2021; Alshawush et al. 2020; Hussein et al. 2017)
4. **Role clarity** (Karkkola et al. 2019; ICN 2020; Klein et al. 2020a; Smith et al. 2019; Torrens et al. 2020)

5.5.1   Key Points for Each Environmental Factor

Support
- The work environment (a primary influence)
- Presence and use of preceptors and mentors (or lack of)
- Educational context
  - Graduate education (didactic and clinical)
  - Proper resources for graduate education and clinical practice
  - Post-graduation workplace orientation
  - Physician support
  - Key stakeholder support (faculty, peers, preceptors, family/friends, patients, formal leadership)

Socialization

- The influence of experienced professional role models
- Immersion in a community of practice
- Clinical encounters with patients
- Workplace values
- Educational requirements of the role
- Culture of country
- Culture of the workplace
- Community social values
- Public perceived image and the perspective of women
- Historical and current subordination of nurses to the medical profession
- Workplace organizational structure

Public Image and Cultural Perspective of Nursing

A country's cultural perspective of the role and function of the nurse develops over time becoming embedded in culture. The patient-nurse relationship, and thus patient care is deeply influenced by the public's perceived status of nursing and women. The effective use of the nurse to work at their full scope, knowledge and ability can be limited by the healthcare work environment that restricts autonomous nursing practice due to the cultural perspective of nursing combined with the community's public image of nursing (Ndirangu, Sarki, Mbekenga & Edwards, 2021; Sheer & Wong, 2008).

APN Role Clarity can be improved by

- A country's stated APN scope of practice
- Formal leadership support and knowledge of the APN role
- Physicians' understanding of the APN role and scope of practice
- Nurses and staff understanding of the APN role and scope of practice
- The population of the country and the people's understanding of the APN role and scope of practice
- A correct workplace APN job description
- An appropriate workplace organizational chart placement of the APN

5.6   Self-Concept

Professional identity and self-concept are linked, yet different. A strong self-concept will build a strong professional identity. An APN's self-concept and professional identity to the APN role can impact those around them by representing the highly educated and knowledgeable nurse who can guide, mentor, and lead others (Girvin et al. 2016; Gutierrez and Morais 2017; Johnson et al. 2012).

Recognizing yourself as nurse and advanced practice nurse student is part of the construction of professional identity and self-concept. Role transition can be a challenging time concerning self-concept as you are in an active learning period of your life. Your outward reflection of your deep, personal, internalized process of who you are as an APN is your *professional image* which is the foundation of your professional identity (Pullen 2021).

The internal sense of who you are as a person is the essence of your *self-concept*. This sense of "who are you" develops in early childhood and continues throughout life with the constant self-evaluation of yourself combined with the comparison of the perceived ideal self (Ackerman 2020). The construction of self-concept is multidimensional including how you see yourself physically, emotionally, socially, spiritually, and professionally. Self-concept includes other "self" constructs including self-esteem, self-image, self-efficacy, and self-awareness (Ackerman 2020).

Self-concept The outcome of one's personal thoughts, feelings, and judgment about oneself in multiple dimensions, plus knowing about one's own tendencies, thoughts, preferences and habits, hobbies, skills, and areas of weakness is your *self-concept*. This self-concept becomes your mental representation of your ability and self-efficacy that you can achieve, complete a task, skill or obtain a set of knowledge that shapes how you feel about yourself, other individuals, and your social relationships (Ackerman 2020; Peiffer et al. 2020; Showers et al. 2015).

Self-concept is:

- Learned, not inherent.
- Started in early childhood.
- Influenced by biological and environmental factors.
- Impacted by social interactions (personal, community, and professional relationships and activities) and culture.
- Displayed uniquely with each person.
- Varied from incredibly positive to very negative (usually a mix of positive and negative concepts).
- Multidimensional with emotional, intellectual, functional, and judgmental dimensions.
- Changed with the context and time.
- A primary influence on the individual's life.
- Directly impacted by identities or professional roles.
- Constantly compared with a personal perception of an "ideal self" (Ackerman 2020; Emery et al. 2018; Kantek and Şimşek 2017; Showers et al. 2015).

Professional self-concept Professional self-concept is combination of personal beliefs and values that guide communication, thoughts, actions combined with one's required professional knowledge and skills creating commitment, personal accountability, and a sense of well-being. The APN educational process and the first

APN position are important aspects of the development of a professional self-concept. Nurses who are actively engaged in their nursing roles will have higher levels of professional attitudes and identity (Çöplü and Tekinsoy Kartın 2019). Your professional self-concept reflects the information and beliefs you have about the APN role, nursing values, and APN scope of practice that enhances your sense of professional identity. This self-concept took on its professional attributes the day you were accepted into your graduate education and APN program. Your professional self-concept will continue to develop and change over your entire career (Goliroshan et al. 2021).

Self-esteem The confidence and satisfaction one has with self, talents, and abilities (Ackerman 2020).

Self-efficacy One's self-judgment of their abilities, skills, and knowledge to execute a course of action to gain what is wanted (Ackerman 2020). A strong professional identity is more likely to improve self-efficacy and resiliency to job pressures and demands (Ageiz et al. 2021).

Self-awareness A personal attribute on the conscious awareness of one's own thoughts, feelings, behaviors, and traits (Ackerman 2020).

Examples of positive professional self-concepts include:

- An APN sees self as an intelligent person.
- An APN perceives self as an important member of his community.
- An APN sees self as an excellent peer support.
- An APN thinks of self as a nurturing and caring person.
- An APN views self as a hard-working and competent employee.
- An APN sees self as an autonomous healthcare provider.

Examples of negative professional self-concepts include:

- An APN sees self as slow to understand healthcare concepts.
- An APN perceives self as expendable and a burden on his community.
- An APN sees self as a terrible peer support.
- An APN thinks of self as an unskilled person.
- An APN views self as an incompetent employee.
- An APN sees self as requiring supervision for most skills and decisions.

There are many dimension-specific self-concepts that encompass our self-concept. Some people may be more positive or negative than others, yet each dimension is an important component of what makes us who we are today. Understanding your current self-concept can help you set your goals for the future.

5.6.1 Steps and Activities to Enhance Your Positive Professional Self-Concept

1. Recognize your strengths/successes and give yourself self-praise for what you do well. (Self-praise is not bragging by comparing yourself to others. Self-praise is acknowledging what you do well.)
2. Increase your responsibilities at work (or as a student).
3. Emphasize the positives. Do not shame yourself for mistakes (learn from them).
4. Set realistic goals.
5. Nurture a positive attitude. Make other people feel welcome. Work on your attentive listening skills. Be kind to others.
6. When involved in a traumatic event, recognize the possibilities of a positive outcome using your strengths. Believe in yourself.
7. Build trusting friendships and relationships in both professional and personal spheres. Obtain mentors. Seek feedback.
8. Provide honest and contrastive feedback to others. Give visible support, respect, and celebration to others' achievements.
9. Build strong communication skills.
10. Build your skills, knowledge, and confidence on collaboration and working within teams. Be a mentor for nursing (Ackerman 2020; Emery et al. 2018; Karanikola 2018; Kantek and Şimşek 2017; Peiffer et al. 2020; Goliroshan et al. 2021; Pullen 2021).

As you consider yourself within your professional role as an APN, you are recognizing and acknowledging your personal professional qualities, your standards that you uphold in your care and decisions, your abilities, knowledge, and creativity (Kantek and Şimşek 2017). The combination of your professional self-concept and your graduate education will help build your confidence for a successful APN role transition.

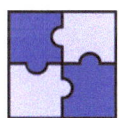

Ways to be proactive in your positive professional self-concept development:

1. Review your APN educational process and recognize your knowledge and skill growth.

_____

_____

_____

2. Nursing performance is based on professional ethics and ethical values. Review the core values of nursing (honesty, altruism, human dignity, autonomy, respect, and social justice) and determine your personal attachment to each value.

Honesty: _____

Altruism: _____

Human Dignity: _____

Autonomy: _____

Respect: _____

Social Justice: _____

3. Write at least three APN skills that you feel you do well

_____

_____

_____

_____

4. Write at least three knowledge areas that you feel you understand very well and will impact your ability to make clinical decisions.

_____

_____

_____

_____

5. Describe a clinical experience where you helped a patient understand their care process.

_____

_____

_____

_____

_____

_____

_____

6. Review your answers to the above five questions and discuss the impact to your professional identity formation.

_____

_____

_____

_____

_____

_____

Clinical decision making is complex and directly impacted by your professional self-concept. Factors involved in clinical decision making include experience, level of education, value of the role played by the professional, area of specialty, chain of command, personal stress, confidence, and beliefs (Farčić et al. 2020). Self-concept can then be impacted by environment and educational processes either subconsciously, or through conscious decisions. Thus, transition from graduate student to APN is a critical point of the career because the theoretical knowledge is placed in context of clinical reality creating abrupt introspection of one's professional self-concept through the required clinical decisions (Farčić et al. 2020). Overall, your professional self-concept will directly impact the care you provide.

> If, as an APN student (or new graduate), you have a sense of responsibility for the APN role, your patients, and yourself, then you will be willing to apply, adapt and expand your knowledge for your patient quickly and properly.

A positive professional self-concept decreases role stress, improves adaptation, decreases burnout, and improves decision-making skills (Goliroshan et al. 2021). The professional self-concept is one of the most important components of health-related professions because it impacts your ability to make clinical decisions, confidence, and enhances the quality of care provided. When you see the APN role as meaningful and it provides valuable activities to help others and you see yourself as becoming an integral part of the role, then you are developing your positive professional self-concept.

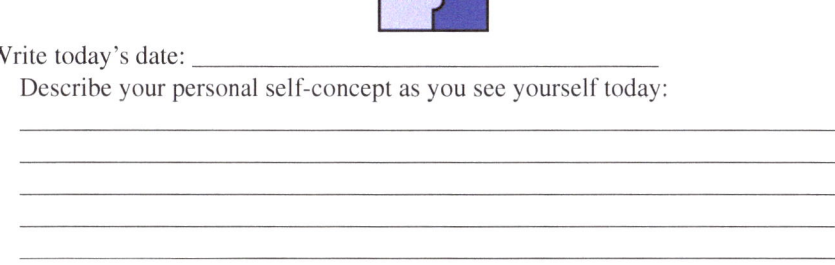

Write today's date: _____

Describe your personal self-concept as you see yourself today:

_____
_____
_____
_____
_____

5.7 Changes in the APN Profession Impacts Professional Identity

A profession itself can change and grow based upon the society's recognition of the profession, the professional values, and the members within that profession (Gutierrez and Morais 2017; Trede 2012). Personal meaning and professional identity grow with the change in the profession's knowledge and skills.

Over the centuries, knowledge and skills have changed in nursing as science has expanded the understanding of health and illness. Nursing has gone from keeping patients clean, fed, and cared for (based on science by nurse Florence Nightingale) to the addition of advanced skills of monitoring complex patients with critical thinking based on knowledge of advanced pathophysiology and the technical skills required to provide the needed care. Nurses are making a difference globally and this drives a change in nursing knowledge and professional identity. Just as every profession has a group of social norms, roles, values, and identity so does every professional has a personal professional identity defining who they are as a person and how they fit within their profession. The identity of nursing is based on the set of knowledge and practices nurses do worldwide. Preparation to join a workforce in a specific profession includes the required profession's knowledge and skills as well as the ability to work in a team, communicate with others, and socializing within the workplace culture through the understanding and incorporation of a professional identity (Trede 2012).

5.7.1 Example of How Increased Knowledge Changed Nursing

The stethoscope was invented in 1816 as a physician's tool (https://www.adctoday.com/learning-center/about-stethoscopes/history-stethoscope). As the technology changed to improve the stethoscope so did the skills and knowledge to use the stethoscope as an important diagnostic tool. Now nurses and APNs around the world use the stethoscope combined with their cardiopulmonary and gastroenterology knowledge to impact care decisions and save lives daily.

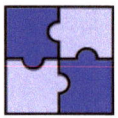

List a few favorite skills or activities that identify you as "Nurse":

_____
_____
_____
_____
_____

Explain how new knowledge impacts the skills or activity over the years:

_____
_____
_____
_____

Although you are in early formation of your APN identity, you can apply future changes to your current professional identity development. Consider the following questions:

How do caring relationships promote health, healing, and effective communication and collaboration?

_____
_____
_____

_____
_____
_____

How, then, does your change in clinical knowledge and skills impact your professional identity through communication with staff and patients?

_____
_____
_____
_____
_____
_____

How does patient-centered care ensure safe, quality patient care and promote the achievement of positive patient outcomes?

_____
_____
_____
_____
_____
_____

How, then, does your patient's outcomes impact your professional identity?

_____
_____
_____
_____
_____
_____

It will be relevant for you to consider your development of your self-concept and personal professional identity every 3–4 months while you are in a graduate program (especially after clinical practicums) or traumatic events/dilemmas because your knowledge and skills are changing rapidly. You should:

- Consciously consider your need for (and obtain) mentors (see Chap. 4).
- Review your self-understanding of right and wrong, your understanding of what it means to be an APN to self, organization, profession, community, country, and world.
- Journal (write) about your role transition, educational experiences, impactful people and events to clarify your self-reflection and understanding who you are becoming (self-concept and professional identity).

You are a nurse and will always have a professional identity as a nurse. You will now need to gain a professional identity as an APN with the expanded nursing role, responsibility, accountability, and authority. The development of your identity as an APN is crucial to provide you confidence, self-resiliency, and internal self-support as you confront barriers and have a successful role transition.

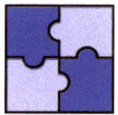

Write today's date: _____

Write about your current attachment and desires of the APN role, what is your current APN professional identity? Are there steps you can take to help you develop a strong APN professional identity?

_____
_____
_____
_____
_____
_____
_____

5.8   Impact of Professional Identity Via Role and Role Transition Stress

Emotion and role stress are entwined together. Role stress can be a physical or psychological strain felt by a student when there is a perception of a lack of ability or resources for the student to perform the role (Sun et al. 2016). Role stress increases when the expectations of the experience are different than the actual experience and achievement. Role stress can occur with:

- Incompatible role expectations
- Too much work is expected to be completed in too little time available
- Vague role expectations without clear paths or support
- Assumptions of perfection being required
- Uncertainty to actual role expectations in clinical practice
- Lack of clear role definition
- Differences between academic and the real-world application of theory with added ethical dilemmas
- Coordination of patients, clinical instructors, and the educational program's expectations
- Role ambiguity and role incompatibility in the workplace
- Lack of support from nursing, administration, peers, or physicians
- Organizational culture that does not support APN (Jones 2014; Sun et al. 2016; ten Hoeve et al. 2014; Woo et al. 2019)

Role stress is an indicator of future burnout and decrease engagement to either the education process or to the final APN role (Sun et al. 2016). Professional identity is the strongest predictor within one's personal characteristics of a student's role stress level. As one develops a stronger professional identity one gains more self-resiliency and lower role stress (Cruess 2006; Johnson et al. 2012; Sun et al. 2016).

The APN role transition is marked by the shift from an experienced, expert status in the generalist nurse role to an inexperienced novice status in the APN role. An unprepared new APN may have experiences that decrease confidence resulting in a decline of self-concept and shift of professional identity. This shift creates role transition stress (Barnes et al. 2021). You will be entering the APN work environment that worldwide is characterized by nursing shortages, increasing patient acuity, and decreasing resources limiting access to healthcare (Hussein et al. 2017). Thus, your role transition will impact your perceptions of nursing, the APN role, your self-concept, professional identity, and self-efficacy. Yet, you can be successful through knowledge and skills acquisition associated with the APN role, role transition process, recognition of barriers and facilitators, and understanding yourself. It is critical to know that as a new APN graduate you will have the cognitive ability, knowledge, and skills to enter the clinical practice workplace. You will continue to learn and grow in the APN role throughout your career as knowledge and technology changes.

To recognize the importance of a successful role transition for new APNs, it is meaningful to understand the potential clinical environment. The APN clinical environment is more complex than the generalist nursing environment. As a generalist nurse you have experienced many common stressors related to the profession: long work hours, dealing with pain, loss and emotional suffering, caring for dying patients, providing support to families, staffing shortages, increasingly complex patients, decreasing resources, and the increased need for knowledge of ever-changing technology (Botha et al. 2015). The APN clinical environment adds the complexity of being a healthcare provider. There are additional changes in the working relationships with increased responsibility and accountability and increased complexity of critical thinking of your assessments, diagnosis, plans, and evaluations with clinical expertise to nurses, physicians, formal leadership, patients, and all stakeholders.

According to Barnes et al. (2021) there are three common domains impacting role transition which are directly connected to your professional identity formation. Each domain is impacted by your personal choices:

1. Educational preparedness
   (a) It is your decision on how you study and obtain knowledge and skills.
   (b) It is your decision to seek help when needed.
2. Role acquisition with subdomains role ambiguity, self-confidence, perceived competence, and mentorship
   (a) It is your decision whether you will be active in gaining self-insight and proactively building your self-concept, self-efficacy, and APN professional identity.
   (b) It is you decision to develop healthy coping mechanisms.
   (c) It is you decision to build your personal support people to share successes and help in times of stress.

3. Job satisfaction with subdomains professional autonomy, quality of professional and interpersonal relationships, time to complete work, job benefits, sense of meaning, and work–life balance. Job satisfaction can take months to fully appreciate and develop.

   (a) Support and positive experiences will provide a positive professional identity.
   (b) It is your decision to gain knowledge and skills to recognize and overcome barriers.
   (c) It is our decision to seek help and support when barriers threaten to overwhelm you.

Supporting novice APNs directly enhances the patient experience and the effectiveness and efficiency of care while building the APNs confidence, knowledge, skills, and professional identity (Barnes et al. 2021).

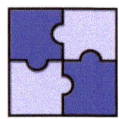

Review the three domains that will impact your role transition and professional identity. Choose at least two aspects and write how you can positively impact yourself and improve your role transition process:

_____
_____
_____
_____
_____
_____

5.9   Barriers

Care related to global healthcare needs is complex. There is a persistent need to provide care to people who live in geographical isolation, political turmoil, cultural disparities (poverty, age, disease), and now a pandemic (Smith et al. 2019; Torrens et al. 2020). Nursing is the largest healthcare professional group. The APN role and scope of practice has the potential to be responsive to the needs of communities and population. The APN provides safe, high-quality care to those in need in many countries. There are barriers and facilitators to APN role implementation and the individual APN role transition process. Many barriers and facilitators of APN role implementation involve professional judgment, working autonomously, and interprofessional and intraprofessional relationships (Torrens et al. 2020). It is important to analyze common barriers APNs face worldwide. It is through acknowledgement that these barriers exist that APNs can develop skills to decrease the effect of barriers.

Workplace staff and lines of responsibility are the two most cited barriers to the implementation of the APN role in the Torrens et al. (2020) scoping review. This includes APNs experiencing team members who would withhold or refuse to share information, decline referral, and place undo restrictions on the APN's responsibilities. Barriers increased when the APN role and scope was not clearly defined especially in relationship to the other team members. Lack of support or understanding of the APN role and scope of practice by administration dramatically increase the barriers and difficulties implementing the APN role successfully (Torrens et al. 2020).

Major barriers that you may encounter are divided into four levels of source impact:

- Macro barriers—barriers from laws, regulations, and economy
- Meso barriers—barriers from your workplace
- Micro barriers—barriers that are found in day-to-day activities
- Self-imposed role transition barriers

Macro barriers: perceived legal, regulatory, and economic barriers

- Nursing roles that are dependent upon your country context, culture, and public perception of nurses
- Lack of APN positions due to lack of understanding role and abilities of the APN
- Scope of practice dependent upon legal and regulatory issues
- Insurance/payment process for APN is often different than for physicians
- Lack of medication prescription authority
- Inadequate funding for NP positions
- Country's current financial abilities and state of health (famine, wars, political strife, weather trauma, housing, water, electricity, food sources)

Meso barriers: local institutional and/or community issues

- Lack of stakeholder support, or overt blocking
- Budget constraints (NPs are paid more than nurses)
- Lack of awareness of the APN role and scope of practice
- Lack of understanding of the role to local leadership, staff, and patients
- Unclear career pathways within the workplace
- Lack of peer or management support
- Team factors creating poor communication or work relationships
- Lines of responsibilities
- Heavy staff workload
- Time demands

Micro Barriers: day-to-day practice environment

- Lack of role clarity/role ambiguity
- Work isolation (working without other APNs or working as the only provider)

- Vertical and lateral othering (passive aggressive and aggressive behavior)
- Professional jealously and perceived threats to role distinction
- Resistance to NP model
- Often higher resistance from nursing
- High workloads
- Improper payment for APN work
- Lack of recognition and use of the APN competencies
- Role conflicts by the addition of responsibilities outside of scope
- Lack of autonomy

Self-placed barriers: Transition stressors

- Unanticipated personal response when involved with death and dying as the provider
- Personal fear of dying due to pandemic
- Uncertainty concerning treatment and lack of confidence
- Conflict with other nurses (see "Bullying")
- Workload with too many patients, or too complex patients for entry into clinical practice
- Conflict with physicians
- Lack of staff support
- Perceived inadequate clinical preparation during the graduate APN education (Alnuqaidan et al. 2021; Faraz 2019; Jones 2014; Klein et al. 2020b; Smith et al. 2019; Torrens et al. 2020; Woo et al. 2019)

Developing your professional identity and a self-concept construction is particularly susceptible to change during times of stress (Emery et al. 2018; Wood and Olivier 2004). Role stress, traumatic events, a poor performance, missed diagnosis, a missed skill, or receiving negative feedback can impact self-concept and professional identity formation. However, almost every APN student will experience a negative event during their educational process. As a graduate student, it is advantageous to study potential barriers that can create negative events to be prepared and minimize the negative impact to self.

Most APNs will experience some barriers. These barriers will decrease your ability to become to reach your potential. Role stress can occur from simple lack of knowledge to overt passive aggressive acts and preplanned barriers. It is imperative to understand the possible barriers so you can recognize barriers and develop skills to overcome stressful events. Below are six common barriers that can be found in the meso, micro, and self-levels:

5.9.1 Role Ambiguity

Role ambiguity occurs when formal workplace leadership, healthcare providers, other nurses, or policy decision makers do not have a clear understanding of the APN scope of practice or role (Gutierrez and Morais 2017; Karanikola et al. 2018;

Klein et al. 2020a; Thompson 2019; Vaismoradi et al. 2011). Role ambiguity can also occur when the APN and other stakeholders hold different viewpoints and understanding of the APN role responsibility, accountability, and authority (Jones 2014). Different viewpoints can be related to the understanding of the scope of practice, traditional viewpoint of nursing and women in your country (Sheer and Wong 2008; ten Hoeve et al. 2014). In countries where the perception of the nurse is "handmaiden to the physician" creates assumptions that block the understanding that APNs (and nurses) are educated to deal with complex health and wellness problems autonomously (ten Hoeve et al. 2014).

Common areas of lack of understanding include:

- Your role in providing care
- Your scope of practice
- The skills you can perform
- Your level of decision-making
- The level of APN autonomy (Woo et al. 2019)

APNs may experience role ambiguity from:
- Patients and patient's family members
- Physicians and healthcare staff
- Supervisors and senior leadership
- The APN's personal friends and family
- Stakeholders and government officials

Different opinions and expectations can impede the extent to which the ANP role can be implemented or expanded. A well-designed response can assist you in describing the APN, the role, scope of practice, authority, and potential benefits of APNs. This information can possibly be gained from your job description.

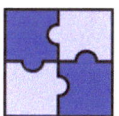

Activity This activity will help you build an effective response to questions people may ask to clarify of the APN role.

Answer the following questions and then write a statement that explains what the function, capabilities, and responsibilities of APNs.

Describe your role as an APN or what you expect your role to be. _____

_____

_____

_____

_____

Describe what your role as APN in the interprofessional relationship between APN and physician. _____

_____

_____

_____

What is the difference between an APN and generalist nurse? _____

_____

_____

_____

Write your answer "I am an APN, which means… _____

_____

_____

_____

_____

_____."

5.9.2   Failure to Complete Introspective Self-Exploration

This book has placed emphasis on self-reflection and introspective exploration as critical components to understanding the complexities of self and to the construction of your APN professional identity. It is essential to understand yourself as person and as a nurse to develop a strong self-concept and professional identity. Critical and creative thinking with ethical decision-making processes are embedded within your personal values, beliefs, attitudes, and past experiences. These past experiences require introspective review with consideration of the outcome, process, and responses to past events that have created past habits and can help create future habits. Self-doubt, high anxiety, and lack of confidence are emotions that are driven by negative thoughts about self and future (Bandura 2018; Wood and Olivier 2004). Utilizing mental preparedness through prospective reflection to look at the future and realize your desired future can provide direction and coherence to your plans and assist in overcoming your fears (Bandura 2018).

> The primary barrier of failure to complete an introspective review is yourself! Remember your professional development is 100% your responsibility and 0% of your mentors and supporters.

> **Self-reflection**
> Self-reflection is an essential tool for role transition. It is the process where you explore and make sense about an experience and then incorporate your decision into your life's paradigm (Baker 2021). Utilizing self-reflection processes can help you gain personal insight as you take into account your

previous nursing knowledge and incorporate new knowledge to improve your critical thinking and decision-making (Mlinar Reljić et al. 2019). A self-reflection journal (writing) is a well-established process to increase nurse's ability to contextualize and understand complex clinical situations (Markman and McMullen 2003; Mlinar Reljić et al. 2019; Pai 2016).

Self-reflection can be accomplished through writing your experiences in a journal, diary, or this book. Self-reflection and insight can also be gained through small discussion groups, or in formal post-clinical explorations. All use a similar process. The Gibbs' reflective cycle was developed by Graham Gibbs in 1988 to give structure to learning from experiences. The process of Gibbs' reflective cycle encourages the person to:

1. Consider a past event that produced strong emotions, then describe the experience
2. Review your feelings and thoughts about the experience
3. Evaluate the experience, both good and bad aspects
4. Analyze the experience from today's perspective to make sense of the situation and how you could change the outcome if a similar experience was present
5. Make a conclusion about what you learned and what you could have done differently
6. Design an action plan for how you would deal with similar situations in the future, or general changes you might find appropriate.

A self-reflection process is particularly helpful to find your hidden clues about consistent personal reaction to negative events, such as negative feedback or passive aggression. Take time to review several past events and determine a plan on how you want to respond in the future.

An excellent website to review and practice self-reflection is:

https://www.ed.ac.uk/reflection/reflectors-toolkit/reflecting-on-experience/gibbs-reflective-cycle

5.9.3 Vertical Discounting

This occurs when a person above or below you in your APN role refuses to recognize your full scope of practice. Often vertical discounting occurs when generalist or specialty nursing staff hold a negative view of the APN role and feel the role has moved away from traditional nursing (Anderson et al. 2020). This discounting and jealousy are usually intentional, and the result can undermine the APN's authority to prescribe treatment plans. Nursing staff may refuse to follow the APNs prescribed orders stating all orders must come from a physician (Jones 2014).

Vertical discounting can also come from above where supervisors or physicians refuse to allow the APN to practice to their full scope of practice and prefer to keep the APN in what they view is a traditional nursing role (Anderson et al. 2020; Jones 2014). This type of vertical discounting is rarely unintentional and often occurs due to lack of knowledge and trust.

The vertical discounting barrier is disheartening to say the least. The first step in overcoming this barrier is not to react, but to respond. A great way to start your response is to ask the person about their perspective of the APN role and seek to understand their thoughts and fears. Then build a response from your understanding of the scope of practice, country context/culture, regulations, and research that support the safe, high-quality care that APNs provide around the world.

Exemplar

Franziska was an APN who was in the process of gaining additional cardiology education to specialize in cardiology to ultimately improve the access to cardiology services to her community. She saw a 58-year-old female who presented with a cold foot that had pallor and no palpable pulses. She immediately reached out to the collaborating cardiologist. He agreed to the circulation compromised and asked Franziska to register the patient for vascular surgery the following day. Franziska completed the patient education with rationale of the diagnosis and plan for surgery. The patient agreed. However, the following afternoon the patient called Franziska concerned with increasing pain and informed Franziska that the physician did not arrive to the hospital to perform the surgery. Franziska contacted the cardiologist who informed her he had an emergency and would perform surgery the following day. Unfortunately, the patient arrived at the clinic the following afternoon in severe pain and reported the physician did not show. Immediately Franziska attempted to contact the cardiologist; however, he was unavailable. She then contacted another vascular surgeon who took the patient immediately to surgery and saved the woman's foot. The next day during the cardiology clinic Franziska's collaborating cardiologist yelled at her in front of staff and patients that she had no right to call another physician and no knowledge of cardiology because she was "just a nurse." He then said, "APNs are stupid."

This vertical abuse was intentional, loud, and public. Franziska knew she could not respond at the time because her collaborating cardiologist was angry and almost violent. She was also uncertain how to respond. Silence was effective in this situation as the physician returned later to apologize. However, she did report the incident because vertical othering should not be tolerated under any circumstances. More importantly she learned that she did have a strong professional identity to the APN role and knew her action was ethical, fit her values, and saved the patient's foot.

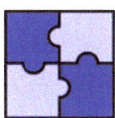

Can you think of a time where you received vertical abuse in the past? Recognition of vertical abuse and understanding the emotional impact can help you prepare to effectively respond to future abuse.

_____
_____
_____
_____
_____

5.9.4 Lateral Othering

When bullying occurs among the same level of professionals, it is called lateraling others (Anderson et al. 2020). This type of barrier comes from someone with your same level of responsibility, accountability, and authority: one APN to another APN creates negative behavior (ambivalence, the silent treatment, bullying, or passive aggressive behavior). Lateral othering is also detrimental to one's confidence and successful transition. The first step in overcoming this barrier is to complete an introspective self-review on past experiences when you were bullied to understand your emotions. Then seek to understand why the person has bullied you (or other negative behaviors). To overcome lateral othering requires a well-planned discussion started in a positive way.

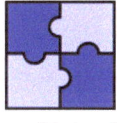

Think of a time when you experienced lateral othering. How did you respond?

_____
_____

In learning to respond to lateral abuse, it is key to understand that the majority of lateral abuse is from jealously and lack of understanding. Seeking to understand the abuser's point of view can aid in ending lateral abuse.

Write at least two actions you will do if you receive lateral othering from another APN.

_____
_____
_____
_____
_____
_____

5.9.5   Work-Family Imbalance

When a person spends too much time at work (or in university), an imbalance between work/university requirements and family needs can occur. Work-family imbalance contributes to increased emotional stress and decreased work engagement (Klein et al. 2020a). This imbalance can be caused by the family's feelings of abandonment related to time requirements of a graduate program and work, or feelings of anger and fear as there is a change in family income dynamics. Overcoming work-balance barriers requires support and discussions with your family to develop a mutually agreed plan. This plan requires an open discussion, plus recognition that it is healthy to have a well-balanced life between work, family, and relaxation.

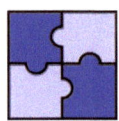

Review your current work-family imbalance. Although you are busy with your advanced education, what short activities could you do with family members?

_____
_____
_____

5.9.6   Shortage of Resources

To be an effective APN, you will need to have resources (equipment, staff, supplies, and funding). Shortage of resources includes all aspects that can impede APN role implementation in your workplace. Problems can arise when there are shortages in appropriate accommodations, nursing staff, appropriate funding, administrative support (including technology), and resources for research and education are withheld from APNs simply because they are an APN (Jones 2014; Woo et al. 2019). These shortages can impact patient care, professional development, and personal morale (Jones 2014). The workplace culture (such as the importance of the nursing role, women, or other disparities that can be aimed at nursing and APN), public perceptions, and social support can directly impact the availability of resources for APNs (Jones 2014; ten Hoeve et al. 2014). Occasionally resources are withheld with a plan to discourage or bully the APN. This is passive aggression. This is a workplace barrier. The important understanding is that as an APN you are a needed healthcare provider and you should receive the same resources as physicians.

Table 5.1 provides five different aspects concerning workplace bullying (victim attributes, perpetrators, common tactics, workplace involvement, and common consequences of bullying). To increase self-resiliency, one should understand the tactics others may use when there is jealousy, anger, fear, or misunderstanding. Thus, understanding Table 5.1 can help you develop predetermined responses for bullying that may occur towards you.

Table 5.1 Workplace bullying

Process	Result
Common victim attributes	• Being new on the job • Having received a promotion • In a new role • Having relationship difficulties • Appearance of receiving special attention from physicians • Working in understaffed conditions • Being young • Being male if in a female-dominated workplace
Common perpetrators	• Nurse: Female with 11 years of experience • Any supervisor, leadership • Physician
Common bullying tactics	• Gossiping • Verbal abuse • Blaming the person for mistakes • Boycotting opportunities (not helping or withholding information). For APNs this includes nurses refusing to follow APN orders • "Tough love" (no support provided with a traumatic situation) • "Sink-or-swim" (forcing a person to work without support or guidance) • Ignore opinions of the victim • Being forced to work below one's competence • Work interference (preventing the person from getting their work done)
Institutional involvement	• A historic prevalence of nurse-to-nurse bullying is tolerated by many workplaces. The chronic, worldwide nursing profession habit of "nurses eat their young" (which means it is alright to bully new nurses and occurs so often it is tradition) remains tolerated and used as a mean of establishing authority over new nurses. • For nurses, 25% of violence is lateral and 75% is vertical by people in higher position of power. • In many workplaces, the leaders minimize complaints creating the culture that reporting bullying may result in retaliation
Consequences	• Feelings of humiliation • Lack of sense of safety at work • Feelings of undervalued • Low self-esteem and impact to self-concept • A shift in professional identity • Loss of sleep, nightmares • Long-term mental health problems: anxiety, guilt, anger, shame, self-blaming, depression, sleep disorders, PTSD • Unhealthy response with gossiping, putdowns, and blaming back to perpetrator or other new employees • Medical errors (with 30% resulting in death) • Unsuccessful role transition, role failure, or transition shock
References	Alshawush et al. (2020), Anderson et al. (2020), Fink-Samnick (2015), Jones (2014), Vidal-Alves et al. (2021)

Bullying
Unfortunately, healthcare settings are common workplaces with a high prevalence of bullying in nursing professions (Alshawush et al. 2020). This bullying is primarily vertical and lateral violence with new and younger professionals receiving more bullying. In 2008, a 10-European-country study found 21% of nurses received harassment from superiors with new nurses with male nurses at higher risk of receiving bullying (Vidal-Alves et al. 2021). The pandemic has increased physical exhaustion, feelings of being at risk for contracting a potential lethal disease and being exposed to highly emotional demanding situations which has escalated workplace bullying in the healthcare workplaces (Vidal-Alves et al. 2021). Nearly 60% of new nurses leave their job due to vertical or lateral abuse (Vidal-Alves et al. 2021).

5.9.7 Physical Assault

Another possibility of workplace violence is actual physical assault. Healthcare providers are at risk for assault which is often described as "part of the job" (Fink-Samnick 2015). One United States study in 2013 reported 76% of nurses with more than 10 years of experience reported at least some sort of assault from patients or visitors (Fink-Samnick 2015). Physical assaults can also come from physicians, such as surgeons throwing surgical tools at nurses when angry in the operating room. Although many healthcare workplaces are under extreme stress due to the pandemic and current economic situation in 2021, that does not make it acceptable to allow violence to persist within the healthcare setting.

5.9.8 Coping Mechanisms

Most nurses will receive some form of bullying or workplace violence. That does not justify the prevalence within workplaces. However, the understanding that one might receive bullying demands that you assess your personal coping mechanisms, so you are prepared to respond in a positive fashion emotionally and professionally. Table 5.2 provides you with common reactions to personal attacks of bullying. Your response can be positive or negative and are often a rapid response based on personal past experiences of similar events. To modify your response to a positive coping response requires you to understand positive responses and predetermine how you will respond when a situation arises.

Table 5.2 Coping mechanisms for abuse

Positive coping mechanisms	Negative coping mechanisms
Active acknowledgment and communication (Help me understand why you are treating me this way? In what way have I offended you?)	Acceptance by self-blaming
	Depression
Religious coping (prayer and forgiveness)	Fear
Positive reinterpretation and growth	Suppression competing activities
Planning responses	Mental disengagement @ workplace
Seeking emotional support	Focus on venting emotions—bullying back/revenge
Restraint to retaliate	Denial
Self-review and validation of knowledge and skills	Anger
Humor (if well planned)	Behavioral disengagement
Know the proper reporting process	Not discussing with person
Report all abuse	Not reporting
Active support of healthy workplace culture activities	Ignoring abuse witnessed to others
	Transferring anger and fear to other people
	Stress eating/smoking/alcohol

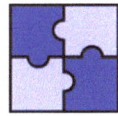

Review the above coping mechanism and consider your past episodes with stressful situations. Write at least two positive coping mechanisms you will use if you are in a bullying situation.

_____

_____

_____

5.10 Facilitators

You have the ability to develop strong personal skills that will provide you with the knowledge and confidence to overcome barriers. You have learned about role transition and role responsibilities, the importance of clear job descriptions, potential barriers, how to identify stakeholders, leadership skills to build self-confidence and self-resiliency, plus education on communication and relationships building and maintenance. Role conflicts can arise from nursing staff, auxiliary staff, physicians, and workplace formal leadership when there is role ambiguity related to lack of understanding of the full scope of practice of the APN (Thompson 2019). Take time to understand and develop skills that will facilitate your successful role transition and development of a positive professional APN identity. Those skills can help you overcome both personal and environmental factors that could become barriers.

5.10.1 Personal Factors

The personal factors that impact role transition to the APN profession within yourself and include:

- Personal coping mechanisms
- Self-awareness preparations (use of self-reflection and forethought)
- Personal motivation and self-resiliency
- Self-efficacy
- Self-concept
- Developing a positive APN professional identity

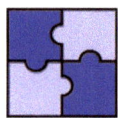

Review the incactivities, you can use to impact the APN facilitators

Personal factor	Activities I can do to promote these personal factors
Coping mechanisms	
Self-awareness preparations (use of self-reflection and forethought)	
Personal motivation	
Self-efficacy	
Self-concept	
Developing an APN professional identity	

The environmental factors that can be facilitators and impact your role transition include:

- A positive workplace environment (culture and organizational structure)
- APN role support (including orientation and mentorships)
- A high level of collaboration or networking available to the APN
- Professional APN organizational involvement (local, national, or international level)
- Interpersonal and interprofessional role clarity
- Adequate preparation for impending role conflicts

- Well-written job descriptions and scope of practice (Branch and George 2017; Hernandez et al. 2017; Roberto 2011; Thompson 2019; Trede 2012; Vaismoradi et al. 2011)

The first job that an APN takes after graduation is a fundamental experience that shapes professional self-concept, resiliency, and professional identity. Interestingly, a 2020 scoping review (Torrens et al. 2020) reports the top two facilitators to implementing the APN role in primary care settings (both clinic and acute care) are team factors and personal factors which were also the top barriers to practice.

- **Team factors** of intra- and interprofessional relationships and working environments can either be supportive or detrimental to the APN.
- **Personal factors** of self-concept, self-efficacy, self-resiliency, and professional identity can either facilitate or be a barrier to the APN successful integration into work process.

Teams that develop strong trust relationships, good communication, have knowledge of the APN role, and scope of practice develop culture to help implement new APNs into primary care settings. The personal factors facilitating successful role transition involve clinical practice, leadership and management skills, use of the APN knowledge competencies, time management, and relationship building and collaboration skills (Torrens et al. 2020).

As with barriers, facilitators are present at the different levels of impact including macro, meso, micro, personal, and orientation/transition programs. A common outcome once APNs were successfully implemented into the workplace, there was improved workplace culture, job satisfaction and retention (Smith et al. 2019).

Macro Facilitators are positive influences or outcomes as a result of legal, regulatory, and economical influence.

- A clearly defined APN role on the legislative and regulatory level
- A well-defined scope of practice with autonomous practice
- Support for graduate education and regulatory endorsement
- National/state health service policy and accreditation
- Adequate funding of APN positions (APN positions should be higher paying than generalist or specialized nursing positions)

Meso Facilitators are positive influences or outcomes of the APN role as a result of the workplace or community.

- Support of APNs with excellent role explanation throughout workplace
- Establishment of formal and informal professional networks for consulting
- Trust relationships
- Understanding and support from formal leadership and managers
- An accurate APN role description to improve clear role understanding
- Proper placement in the organizational structure (if organization structure is used)

- Clear career pathway
- Established transition to practice or formal workplace orientation programs for APNs

Micro Facilitators are day-to-day positive impacts of the APN to the act of providing healthcare to the local community.

- Recognition of the knowledge, skills, and capabilities of the APN to provide high-quality and safe care
- Support for continual learning and professional development
- Development of interprofessional teamwork
- Support from the patients and their families
- Using professional judgment to build trust and provide safe, high-quality care
- Support and encourage APNs to work autonomously
- Interpersonal and intrapersonal relationships
- Strong clinical leadership skills
- Mentorship and role-modeling

Personal facilitators are positive impacts that you do for yourself

- Have an excellent self-incorporation of nursing ethics
- Have an excellent understanding of the APN scope of practice, regulations and role within your country context
- Have an established group of peers, friends, and family for support
- Understand your personal values and leadership style
- Have a mentor (Chap. 4)
- Have reviewed and determined personal responses and process to address passive aggression
- Have developed a plan for personal role transition (Chap. 6)
- Have completed personal reflection and understand the process of professional self-concept and professional identity
- Be responsible and accountable for actions and knowledge
- Able to demonstrate expertise in clinical practice, clinical leadership and management
- Have APN knowledge and skills, and use of evidence-based practices
- Acknowledge good APN educational background by others
- Prior work experiences and previous success in transitions in life and professional settings
- Personal satisfaction with nursing and strong professional identity
- Strong personal ethics and agreement with nursing values and ethics
- Finds meaning in work
- Have a positive work–life balance (Colquitt et al. 2007; Faraz 2019; Goliroshan et al. 2021; Leslie and Lonneman 2016; Smith et al. 2019; Torrens et al. 2020)

Transitional programs are formal workplace programs that provide workplace orientation, mentorship, and ease new APNs into practice. Many workplaces have transitional programs to allow new APNs to have mentorship in making clinical decisions, diagnosis, treatment plans, clinical pharmacology, working in interprofessional and intraprofessional teams, charting, and management skills (especially time). Well-designed programs have proven to help support new APNs through their role transition with improvement in leadership, communication, clinical decisions, and socialization into the workplace (Ageiz et al. 2021; Alshawush et al. 2020; Barnes et al. 2021; Hussein et al. 2021).

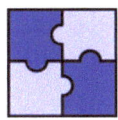

Review the personal factors for facilitators provided above. Choose at least four that you identify as critical to your personal success and briefly write how the identified facilitator will help you as an APN.

_____

_____

_____

_____

_____

_____

_____

_____

5.11 Summary

This chapter provides an in-depth understanding on personal reflections of one's changing professional identity that is deeply impacted by APN graduate education, APN role transition, and clinical practice. There are identified common barriers and facilitators to the APN. This chapter explored the four levels of barriers and facilitators: macro, meso, micro, and self-placed. Within each level, there are activities which can be completed to guide personal forethought and aid a positive role transition and professional identity formation. The top two APN workplace facilitators and the top two APN barriers are the same. Team factors (involving relationships and interpersonal factors) and personal factors (intrapersonal relationship) can be either a facilitator or a barrier. Chapter 7 provides an in-depth discussion on relationships.

References

Ackerman CE (2020) What is self-concept? A psychologist explains. https://positivepsychology.com/self-concept/. Accessed 13 May 2020

Ageiz MH, Elshrief HA, Bakeer HM (2021) Developing a professionalism manual for nurse managers to improve their perception regarding professionalism and professional identity. SAGE Open Nurs 7:23779608211026174. https://doi.org/10.1177/23779608211026174. PMID: 34222656; PMCID: PMC8221667

Alnuqaidan H, Alhajraf A, Mathew P, Ahmad M (2021) Transitional shock of multi-nationality newly graduate nurses in Kuwait. SAGE Open Nurs 7:2377960821998530. https://doi.org/10.1177/2377960821998530. PMID: 33869747; PMCID: PMC8020764

Alshawush KA, Hallett N, Bradbury-Jones C (2020) Impact of transition programmes for students and new graduate nurses on workplace bullying, violence, stress and resilience: a scoping review protocol. BMJ Open 10(10):e038893. https://doi.org/10.1136/bmjopen-2020-038893. PMID: 33127633; PMCID: PMC7604821

Anderson H, Birks Y, Adamson J (2020) Exploring the relationship between nursing identity and advanced nursing practice: an ethnographic study. J Clin Nurs 29:1195–1208. https://doi.org/10.1111/jocn.15155

Baker EL, Murphy SA (2021) A systematic approach to job transitions-Finding your way and landing in the best place. Journal of Public Health Management & Practice 27(1):88–91. https://doi.org/10.1097/PHH.0000000000001231

Bandura A (2018) Toward a psychology of human agency: pathways and reflections. Perspect Psychol Sci 13(2):130–136. https://doi.org/10.1177/1745691617699280

Barlow NA, Hargreaves J, Gillibrand W (2018) Nurses' contributions to the resolution of ethical dilemmas in practice. Nurs Ethics 25(2):230–242. https://doi.org/10.1177/0969733017703700

Barnes H (2015) Exploring the factors that influence nurse practitioner role transition. Journal of Nurse Practitioners. February 11(2):178–183. https://doi.org/10.1016/j.nurpra.2014.11.004

Barnes H, Asefeh Faraz C, Rubright JD (2021) Development of the novice nurse practitioner role transition scale: an exploratory factor analysis. J Am Assoc Nurse Pract 34(1):79–88. https://doi.org/10.1097/JXX.0000000000000566

Bleich M (2017) Job and role transitions: the pathway to career evolution. Nurs Adm Q 41(3):252–257. https://doi.org/10.1097/NAQ0000000000000233

Botha E, Gwin T, Purpora C (2015) The effectiveness of mindfulness based programs in reducing stress experienced by nurses in adult hospital settings: a systematic review of quantitative evidence protocol. JBI Database Syst Rev Implement Rep 13(10):21–29. https://doi.org/10.11124/jbisrir-2015-2380

Branch W, George M (2017) Reflection-based learning for professional ethical formation. Am Med Assoc 19(4):349–356

Cherry K (2020) Introspection in psychology: Wundt's experimental technique. https://www.verywellmind.com/what-is-introspection-2795252

Colquitt JA, Scott BA, LePine JA (2007) Trust, Trustworthiness, and trust propensity: a meta-analytic test of their unique relationships with risk taking and job performance. Journal of Applied Psychology 92(4):909–927. https://doi.org/10.1037/0021-9010.92.4.909

Çöplü M, Tekinsoy Kartın P (2019) Professional self-concept and professional values of senior students of the nursing department. Nurs Ethics 26(5):1387–1397. https://doi.org/10.1177/0969733018761171. Epub 2018 Apr 19. PMID: 29673290

Cruess RL (2006) Teaching professionalism. Clin Orthop Relat Res 449:177–185. https://doi.org/10.1097/01.blo.0000229274.28452.cb

Cruess S, Cruess R, Steinert Y (2019) Supporting the development of professional identity: general principles. Med Teach 41(6):641–649. https://doi.org/10.1080/0142159X.2018.1536260

Emery L, Gardner W, Carswell K, Finkel E (2018) You can't see the real me: attachment avoidance, self-verification, and self-concept clarity. Personal Soc Psychol Bull 44(8):1133–1146. https://doi.org/10.1177/0146167218760799

Faraz A (2019) Facilitators and barriers to the novice nurse practitioner workforce transition in primary care. J Am Assoc Nurse Pract 31(6):364–370. https://doi.org/10.1097/JXX.0000000000000158

Farčić N, Barać I, Lovrić R, Pačarić S, Gvozdanović Z, Ilakovac V (2020) The influence of self-concept on clinical decision-making in nurses and nursing students: a cross-sectional study. Int J Environ Res Public Health 17(9):3059. https://doi.org/10.3390/ijerph17093059. PMID: 32354029; PMCID: PMC7246852

Fink-Samnick E (2015) The new age of bullying and violence in health care. Prof Care Manag 20(4):165–174. https://doi.org/10.1097/NCM.0000000000000099

Girvin J, Jackson D, Hutchinson M (2016) Contemporary public perception of nursing: a systematic review and narrative synthesis of the international research evidence. The Journal of Nursing Management 24:994–1006. https://doi.org/10.1111/jonm.12413

Goliroshan S, Nobahar M, Raeisdana N, Ebadinejad Z, Aziznejadroshan P (2021) The protective role of professional self-concept and job embeddedness on nurses' burnout: structural equation modeling. BMC Nurs 20(1):203. https://doi.org/10.1186/s12912-021-00727-8. PMID: 34666759; PMCID: PMC8524863

Grosemans I, Coertjens L, Kyndt E (2020) Work-related learning in the transition from high education to work: The role of the development of self-efficacy and achievement goals. British Journal of Educational Psychology 90;19–42. https://doi.org/10.1111/blep.12258

Gutierrez MGR, Morais SCRV (2017) Systematization of nursing care in the formation of professional identity. Rev Bras Enferm 70(2):436–442. https://doi.org/10.1590/0034-716-2016-0515

Hernandez PR, Bloodhart B, Barnes RT, Adam AS, Clinton SM, Pollack I et al (2017) Promoting professional identity, motivation, and persistence: benefits of an informal mentoring program for female undergraduate students. PLoS One 12(11):e0187531. https://doi.org/10.1371/journal.pone.0187531

Hussein R, Everett B, Ramjan LM, Hu W, Salamonson Y (2017) New graduate nurses' experiences in a clinical specialty: a follow up study of newcomer perceptions of transitional support. BMC Nurs 16:42. https://doi.org/10.1186/s12912-017-0236-0. PMID: 28775671; PMCID: PMC5534089

International Council of Nursing (2020) Guidelines on advanced practice nursing. Geneva. https://www.icn.ch/system/files/documents/2020-04/ICN_APN%20Report_EN_WEB.pdf. Accessed 17 April 2020

Johnson M, Cowin LS, Wilson I, Young H (2012) Professional identity and nursing: contemporary theoretical developments and future research challenges. Int Nurs Rev 59(11):562–569. https://doi.org/10.1111/j.1466-7657.2012.01013.x

Jones ML (2014) Role development and effective practice in specialist and advanced practice roles in acute hospital settings: systematic review and meta-synthesis. Journal of Advanced Nursing 49(2):191–209

Kantek F, Şimşek B (2017) Factors relating to professional self-concept among nurse managers. J Clin Nurs 26(23–24):4293–4299. https://doi.org/10.1111/jocn.13755. Epub 2017 Mar 28. PMID: 28177549

Karanikola M, Doulougeri K, Koutrouba A, Giannalopoulou M, Papathanassoglou EDE (2018) A phenomenological investigation of the interplay among professional wort appraisal, self-esteem and self-perception in nurses: The revelation of an internal and external criteria system. Frontiers in Psychology 9:1805. https://doi.org/10.3389/fpsyg.2018.01805

Karkkola P, Kuittinen M, and Hintsa T (2019) Role clarity, role conflict, and vitality at work: The role of the basic needs. Scandinavian Journal of Psychology, October 60(5):456–463. https://doi.org/10.1111/sjop.12550

Klein CJ, Weinzimmer LG, Lizer M, Colling M, Pierce L, Dalstrom M (2020a) Exploring burnout and job stressors among advanced practice providers. Nursing Outlook, 68(2):145–154. https://doi.org/10.1016/j.outlook.2019.09.005

Klein C, Weinzimmer LG, Cooling M, Lizer S (2020b) Burnout and job stressors among advanced practice providers. Nurs Outlook 68(2):145–154. https://doi.org/10.1016/j.outlook.2019.09.005

Kline CC, Park SE, Godolphin WJ, Towle A (2020) Professional identity formation: a role for patients as mentors. Acad Med 95(10):1578–1586. https://doi.org/10.1097/ACM.000000000000356

Kowalski K (2019) Mentoring. The Journal of Continuing Education in Nursing 50(12):540–541. https://doi.org/10.3928/00220124-20191115-04

Leslie JL, Lonneman W (2016) Promoting trust in the registered nurse-patient relationship. Home Healthc Now. 34(1):38–42. https://doi.org/10.1097/NHH.0000000000000322. PMID: 26645843

Markman KD, McMullen MN (2003) A reflection and evaluation model of comparative thinking. Personal Soc Psychol Rev 7(3):244–267. https://doi.org/10.1207/S15327957PSPR0703_04

Mlinar Reljić N, Pajnkihar M, Fekonja Z (2019) Self-reflection during first clinical practice: the experiences of nursing students. Nurse Educ Today 72:61–66. https://doi.org/10.1016/j.nedt.2018.10.019

Ndirangu EW, Sarki AM, Mbekenga C, Edwards G (2021) Professional image of nursing and midwifery in East Africa: an exploratory analysis. BMC Nurs 20:37. https://doi.org/10.1186/s12912-020-00531-w

Nocerino R, Chiarini M, Mariana M (2020) Nurse professional identity: validation of the Italian version of the questionnaire nurse professional values scale-revised. Clin Ter 171(2):e114–e119. https://doi.org/10.7417/CT.2020.2200

Pai HC (2016) Development and validation of the simulation learning effectiveness scale for nursing students. J Clin Nurs 25(21–22):3373–3381. https://doi.org/10.1111/jocn.13463. Epub 2016 Aug 31. PMID: 27378308.

Peiffer H, Ellwart T, Preckel F (2020) Ability self-concept and self-efficacy in higher education: an empirical differentiation based on their factorial structure. PLoS One 15(7):e0234604. https://doi.org/10.1371/journal.pone.0234604. PMID: 32692752; PMCID: PMC7373275

Pullen R (2021) Profession identity in nursing practice. Nurs Made Incred Easy 19(2):55–56. https://doi.org/10.1097/01.NME.0000732012.99855.78

Reynolds J, Mortimore G (2021) Transitioning to an ACP: a challenging journey with tribulations and rewards. British Journal of Nursing 30(3):166

Roberto MA (2011) Transformational leadership: how leaders change ream, companies, and organizations. The Great Courses. Chantilly, Virginia

Sheer B, Wong FKYM (2008) The development of advanced nursing practice globally. Journal of Nursing Scholarship 40(3);204–211

Showers CJ, Ditzfeld CP, Zeigler-Hill V (2015) Self-concept structure and the quality of self-knowledge. J Pers 83(5):535–551. https://doi.org/10.1111/jopy.12130. Epub 2014 Oct 30. PMID: 25180616; PMCID: PMC4346517

Smith T, McNeil K, Mitchell R, Boyle B, Ries N (2019) A study of macro-, meso- and micro-barriers and enablers affecting extended scopes of practice: the case of rural nurse practitioners in Australia. BMC Nurs 18:14. https://doi.org/10.1186/s12912-019-0337-z

Sun L et al (2016) The impact of professional identity on role stress in nursing students: A cross-sectional study. International Journal of Nursing Studies 63:1–8. http://dx.doi.org/10.1016/j.ijnurstu.2016.08.010

ten Hoeve Y, Jansen G, Roodbol P (2014) The nursing profession: public image, self-concept and professional identity. A discussion paper. J Adv Nurs 70(2):295–307

Thompson A (2019) An educational intervention to enhance nurse practitioner role transition in the first year of practice. Am Assoc Nurse Pract 31(1):24–32. https://doi.org/10.1097/jxx.0000000000000095

Torrens C, Campbell P, Hoskins G et al (2020) Barriers and facilitators to the implementation of the advanced nurse practitioner role in primary care settings: a scoping review. Int J Nurs Stud 104:103443. https://doi.org/10.1016/j.ijnurstu.2019.103443

Trede F (2012) Role of work-integrated learning in developing professionalism and professional identity. Asia Pac J Coop Educ 13(3):159–167

Vaismoradi M, Salsali M, Ahmadi F (2011) Perspective of Iranian male nursing students regarding the role of nursing education in developing a professional-identity: a content analysis study. Jpn J Nurs Sci 8:174–183. https://doi.org/10.1111/j.1742-7924.2010.00172.x

Vidal-Alves et al (2021) Tough love lessons: lateral violence among hospital nurses. Int J Environ Res Public Health 18(17):9183. https://doi.org/10.3390/ijerph18179183

Wald H (2015) Professional identity formation in medical Education: Reflection. Relationship, Resilience. Academic Medicine 90(6):701–706. https://doi.org/10.1097/ACM.0000000000000731

Walleck C (1991) Building a framework for dealing with ethical issues. AORN J 53(5):1248–1252

Wensel TM (2006) Mentor or preceptor: What is the difference? American Journal of Health-System Pharmacy 63(17):597. https://doi.org/10.2146/ajhp060121

Woo BFY, Zhou W, Lim TW, Tam WWS (2019) Practice patterns and role perception of advanced practice nurses: a nationwide cross-sectional study. J Nurs Manag 27:992–1004. https://doi.org/10.1111/jonm.12759

Wood LA, Olivier MA (2004) A self-efficacy approach to holistic student development. S Afr J Educ 24(4):289–294

Understanding Self: A Personal Guide for Successful Role Transition

6

6.1 Introduction

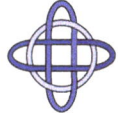

To aspire you must be curious. To achieve your aspiration, you must have a plan. A well-designed plan will guide a successful APN role transition. This chapter will provide you with step-by-step instructions on how to create values, vision, mission, goals, and action plans for a successful personalized role transition plan (PTP). You will gain an understanding of your professional identity through a personal planning process. Understanding self as both person and professional nurse requires an introspective look at yourself to consider your past for habits while considering the future you desire. It is beneficial for you to take time to think about how you plan on becoming a successful APN, overcoming barriers, and using facilitators. Yet, it is instrumental to have a written plan!

6.2 Definitions

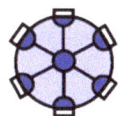

A Strategic Plan A plan that has been made with critical thought and planning for a specific achievement with a disciplined effort to produce fundamental decisions and actions that shape and guide the what, how, and why of actions of a person, team, or organization (Bryson et al. 2018). A strategic plan includes a set of responses concerning the person's values, vision, mission, goals, and action plans.

Definitions of Strategic Plan terms (Williams 2002).

- Values = WHY your behavior/activities are consistent
- Vision = WHAT you want to accomplish
- Mission = HOW to accomplish your vision and to WHOM
- Goals = The "Big Steps" to accomplish your vision
- Action Plans = Specific steps to accomplish your goals with SMART as "I will.." statements. SMART =
  - Specific outcome
  - Measurable
  - Attainable
  - Realistic
  - Time Bond

6.3   What Is a Personal Transition Plan (PTP)?

A personal transition plan is a written document that is developed to clearly state an intended goal of a successful transition from a generalist nurse to a novice APN to an expert APN. When planning involves strategic thinking, you have an integrated and disciplined approach to decision-making while combining short-term and long-term goals to devise a specific plan (Schober 2017). You will be making several strategic decisions as you develop your personalized plan for success.

Completing a personal transition plan (PTP) creates personal empowerment and enhanced engagement to self and professional identity. This process will take time to develop an effective and impactful personal transitional plan. You can review and modify your PTP as you gain knowledge, skills, experience, and confidence for your APN role. A critical step in successful role transition is the act of introspection and forethought; a PTP is an additional step to enhance the success and attainment of your aspirations.

The outcomes of the process of developing a personal transitional plan are to:

1. Establish a vision to strive for every day through your role transition.
2. Establish a set of values that truly reflect who you are and what behaviors you accept.
3. Implement a process to build and engage others to build capacity and trust to achieve a goal.

6.3.1   Personal Transition Plans (PTP) Background

An excellent way to gain a deeper understanding of who you are becoming is to develop a strategic plan that requires you to deeply consider values, vision, and mission statements which reflect your aspirations of future achievements (Garcia 2016). Personal strategic plans can be designed for a lifelong personal aspiration, a short-term personal goal, a personal or work project, or skill/knowledge acquisition. Your personalized transition plan (PTP) will be a specific strategic plan to your APN role transition. Having a clearly written PTP will enable you to achieve APN transition and test new APN skills/knowledge to overcome barriers and use facilitators to build a strong professional self-concept and professional identity for the APN role (see Chap. 5).

Traditionally strategic planning has been used for the development of a product, service line, or organization (Bryson et al. 2018). However, planning for yourself is critical for positive self-concept because you must understand yourself before you can help others. A PTP is remarkably like formal workplace strategic plans. You will identify values, a vision statement, a mission statement, goals on how to achieve your aspiration, and finally action plans on how you will achieve your goals. In the past, personal strategic planning was a process only for formal senior leaders, directors, and chief executive officers (CEOs). Gaining the knowledge and ability to build and implement a PTP will allow you to realize the effectiveness of well-written plans for people working in the clinical setting as well as in formal leadership roles.

If you build a personal strategic plan and say your vision out loud daily, review your values with the decisions that you make, then it is possible to develop a strong self-concept deeply imbedded in integrity. If you develop a personal set of values and a vision statement, but never look at it or use the values to drive your behavior, then your plan becomes merely words on the page. There is a scarcity of literature on the topic of personal strategic plans. Perhaps the scarcity is because it is often difficult to consider yourself in terms of your future aspirations, goals to accomplish, passions that drive you, and values you wish to uphold. This process will take time and requires honest thoughts about yourself.

As an APN, you will be looked upon as an educated nurse leader and role model simply by being an APN. This is part of your increased accountability and responsibility as an APN. This innate responsibility as nurse leader related to your education is a perfect fit to your APN role and responsibilities of educator, collaborator, mentor, and clinical expert. The first step is a successful transition. As has been said, research around the world reports the APN role transition is difficult. Developing and implementing your PTP is an excellent tool to use to facilitate your graduate education, translating didactic knowledge into clinical expertise and providing a guide for you to overcome barriers.

6.3.2   Barriers to Building a Personal Transition Plan

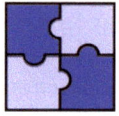

What do you think is the greatest barrier to building a successful strategic plan?

_____

_____

_____

_____

Your greatest roadblock and critic to any of your personal strategic plans will be yourself (Garcia 2016)! Although you are accountable for your own professional growth and success, you will also be the one making excuses or thinking of yourself as a failure. Your success to achieve your aspiration is greatly enhanced if your plan is written down. The main attribute to success is planning. You are an important person right now right at this moment. Now invest in yourself, see your strengths, ponder your future, aspire to do wonderful things, and then build your plans.

6.3.3   Overcoming Yourself as a Barrier

The ability to motivate and guide yourself is using the process of forethought [a planned, premediated process to consider self and future] (Bandura 2018). Forethought allows you to look to the future and realize your desired future to provide you direction and coherence for your plans and to overcome your fears (Bandura 2018).

Steps to overcoming the barrier of yourself:

1. Take time to think about the questions.
2. Be honest, use self-reflectiveness to review challenges in the setting of your skills, abilities, and desires.
3. Consider what you want from your role transition to APN.
4. Complete the preparation work before starting to build your PTP (below).
5. Do not blame others for your failures and barriers.
6. Likewise, do not create barriers for yourself ("I cannot…"). Seek to understand your strengths and creativity and celebrate your courage to try new tasks, processes, knowledge, or skills.

Reviewing self and developing all personal strategic plans are lifelong tasks (Bandura 2018). It is important for you to understand the positive aspects, or gifts, that you possess. In addition, it is difficult, if not impossible, to mentor others to their full potential if we have not looked at ourselves and gained insight related to what drives us and accept our full creative abilities. Developing a PTP is complex, but doable.

Self-Reflection About Self

Perhaps all humans often make comparisons to imagined outcomes, to compare themselves, to their past and future selves, and to other people. As you progress in your role transition from generalist nurse to APN, you will imagine what your new role will be like and how you will accomplish the APN role.

When you are imagining the future, there are typically two concurrent thoughts (Markman and McMullen 2003):

- Reflection = "What if…"
- Evaluation = "How do I compare with others…"

Your thoughts can be positive or negative. When conducting self-reflection take a moment to consider how you are feeling about yourself and the positive activities you are doing in nursing and for your future patients. Role transition is difficult so take time to self-reflect on your journey and talk with other nurses, fellow students, mentors, and instructors to help you on your journey. Seek positive thoughts of who you were and who you are becoming.

An excellent website to review and practice self-reflection is:

https://www.ed.ac.uk/reflection/reflectors-toolkit/reflecting-on-experience/gibbs-reflective-cycle

6.4   Preparation for Developing Your Personal Transition Plan (PTP): Introspection

A personal transition plan (PTP) takes time because you will need to think about your nursing career, educational process, clinical experiences, yourself, your workplace, and your possible future. As with all complex projects, the time taken to prepare for design and implementation is important. You are important, thus taking time to understand your foundation (passion and gifts) will give you additional insight into who you are as a unique person.

6.4.1   Steps for Preparation: Passions, Gifts, and Aspirations

Step 1: Discover Your gifts

The foundation of developing a personal vision is to understand your gifts. Discovering which gifts you believe are most important for your aspiration (in this case, your successful APN role transition) requires that you look at your talents. Remember a gift is defined as "a notable capacity, talent, or endowment" (https://www.merriam-webster.com/dictionary/gifts).

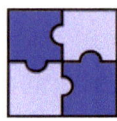

List your talents, strengths, endowments, capacities, or activities you do well and will help you as an APN

_____
_____
_____
_____
_____
_____
_____

Step 2: Determine Your Passion

Passions are activities you love to do and typically are related to your strengths and gifts (talents). Your behavior is directly attached to your values, therefore understanding passions will help clarify values. As humans we have many parts that make us whole: emotionally (what makes you happy), spiritually (what guides you to want to help others), and physically (what makes you healthy). Think about each area and write down what you really like to do now, what you hold is particularly important in your life. "Passion" is what drives us daily; it is what we find happiness in doing every day. What would you do every day if you could… what is your PASSION? You may have more than one! Write down all the aspects of life that you are passionate about. Then circle the primary passions that you think impact you the most.

Think about what you do that makes you happy.

Here are some ideas:

- Daily prayer time
- Friend time and family time
- Reading and learning
- Completing technical projects
- Helping other people
- Teaching others
- My profession
- Artwork
- Designing future ideas
- Exercising
- Learning a language
- Making and implementing excellent podium presentations

Others:_____
_____
_____

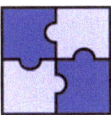

What are your passions? Your gifts? List the activities you love to do? Write down 3–5 items that are your passion or gifts. These are activities that if you do them every day, you would feel great.

_____
_____
_____
_____

Step 3: Determine Your "What I Want to Do/Accomplish"

Everybody wonders about the future and what it might bring for them. Sometimes we envision a project, a degree, a job that we would want to obtain. However, if you only think of your desire as a thought without a plan, you may not get there. What do you want to be doing in three (3) and six (6) months, 1 year and 2–5 years from now concerning your APN role? Write it down! People who write down a goal increase their chance of success by over 40% and if you tell another person about your goal, the success rate is greater than 80%. Unfortunately, most people (about 76%) never write down their goals (Murphy 2018).

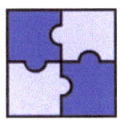

Please take some time and write down some ideas about using your passions and your SWOT analysis (see Step 4) to answer the following question.

3 months from now for my APN role, I would like to:

_____
_____

6 months from now for my APN role, I would like to…_____

_____
_____

1–2 years from now for my APN role, I would like to…

_____

_____

2–5 years from now for my APN role, I would like to … _____

_____

_____

Why Should You Write Down Your Goals?

Let us take a break and return to our physiology of the brain. How did you learn your advanced education? Did you study? Did you take notes? To understand memory encoding, one must understand the interactions of multiple parts of the brain, the environment, and your perceptions. Although not completely understood the frontal lobe, thalamus, amygdala, and hippocampus interact from a perception of a thought to the translation of a memory. The more personally meaningful actions or thoughts are, the more effective encoding. The act of writing down your thoughts concerning your personal transition plan increases the physical activity of the brain and enhances the encoding process, thereby creating a reality frame in your memory (Murphy 2018; The Human Memory. Memory Encoding 2019)

STEP 4: Complete a SWOT Analysis

One strategy to help guide your thoughts is to conduct a SWOT analysis for yourself. "SWOT" stands for Strengths-Weakness-Opportunities-Threats (Teoli and An 2020). A SWOT analysis is typically depicted as a four-quadrant box. If you take time to explore each aspect concerning yourself and your future plan as APN, then you will recognize the strengths and weaknesses you have, the opportunities to help you grow, and the barriers (or threats) so you can make plans to successfully overcome them.

The SWOT analysis has been used for over 60 years as a business tool and has been applied to individual assessments (Teoli and An 2020). It is typically used in business to assess the environment of both internal and external forces from the perspective of every stakeholder. When used for a personal tool, the person completes the SWOT from a personal perspective (von Kodolitsch et al. 2015).

The SWOT is typically divided into internal (or controllable) aspects of strengths and weaknesses and the external aspects (or uncontrollable) of opportunity and threats (Teoli and An 2020). A starting point for a personal role transition SWOT can be using the Barnes concept analysis (2015) antecedents:

Personal Antecedents (controllable aspects) for you to become an APN: graduate-level education, disengagement with the generalist nurse role/work, engagement to APN roles, and a desire for feedback.

Environmental Antecedents (uncontrollable aspects) for you to become an APN: APN Job novelty, support, formal orientation.

Review each antecedent and determine if you have a strength, weakness, opportunity, or threat in achieving each antecedent. Write your thoughts in the SWOT table.

6.4.2 Personal SWOT

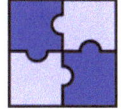

Complete a personal SWOT analysis of yourself. Provide answers where you are currently in your APN role transition and professional identity development. Then you can review the answers to determine if your actions have provided the picture that reflects your vision of your true self. Once you graduate, you should repeat your personal SWOT to provide you guidance and show your increased strengths gain in your APN education. This exercise is a personal SWOT analysis and the table provides you with space to write your responses to the SWOT analysis questions.

6.4.3 Personal SWOT Analysis

Personal **STRENGTHS**—what do you do well? What resources can you draw upon? What do others see as your strengths?

OPPORTUNITIES to you—What opportunities are open to you? What trends, knowledge or skills can you take advantages of? How can you turn your weaknesses into opportunities?

Personal **WEAKNESSES**—What could you improve? Where do you have fewer resources than others? What do others see as your weaknesses?

THREATS to you or because of you or your role—What threats could harm you (mentally, physically, or spiritually)? What weakness can become a threat?

What strengths can help you with your weaknesses or threats? A word about weaknesses & strengths- No person is strong in every activity to complete your job. Almost every person knows his/her weaknesses. Many people examine their weaknesses and then try to find ways to make those areas stronger. Although this can be a great process for some weaknesses, a person can then spend a great deal of time working on weaknesses instead of growing their strengths. Leading by your strengths can help develop your most effective leadership skills (Rath and Conchie, 2008). It is critical that you review and acknowledge your strengths and recognize your weaknesses so you can determine what strength can help offset what weakness. In some cases what you perceive as a weakness may really have a hidden strength_____

_____
_____
_____
_____

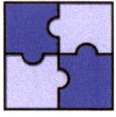

It is wise to understand that some weaknesses are actually opportunities. Review your acknowledged weaknesses. Consider an opportunity that can come about through one of your weaknesses. Write an action or process you can do to address a weakness.

Exemplar
Martin is a shy and quiet young man in his graduate APN education. At his university he has seen many strong leaders that were charismatic, outgoing, and spoke loudly. It was through his personal SWOT assignment that he realized his "weakness" of being quiet was actually an opportunity and strength because he spent time truly listening to people's conversations and was able to propose creative solutions to problems being discussed. Martin is learning that clinical leadership and being a mentor is not dependent on being outgoing, charismatic, or a loudspeaker.

_____
_____
_____
_____
_____

6.4.4   A 360 SWOT

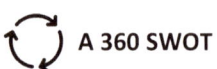 A 360 SWOT

If you want to truly understand yourself, you can ask a few people to also fill a SWOT on you! This is called a 360 SWOT. Listening and understanding what others think of you is powerful and can help you understand yourself and inspire you to reach new levels of clinical leadership. If you ask others, choose your people wisely, and explain that honest answers must be provided. Some people to consider would be a trusted peer, a mentor, a friend, valued instructor, or a wise family member.

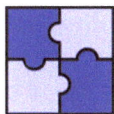

To conduct a 360 SWOT, print a blank SWOT and give it to your chosen people (or via email) and ask for a return in 3–5 days.

> You are now ready to start the personal exploration and building processes of your personal transition plan.

A personal transition plan (PTP) takes time because you will need to think about your ideas of the APN role, about yourself, your workplace, your past, and your possible future.

- Take time to write down your thoughts, because once you write them down, you can acknowledge your thoughts as real possibilities.
- Remember **every idea is important,** so write them down.
- There are five main steps to accomplish:
  - Choose your personal values
  - Develop your strong personal vision statement (what you aspire to accomplish)
  - Complete the process of achievement through your mission statement
  - Develop goals that are the obtainable big steps to achieve your vision
  - Determine the action plans that enable you to easily obtain your goals

6.5   Step 1: Building Your PTP—Values

> **Values are the WHY something is done!**

6.5.1   Background on Personal and Professional Values

VALUES directly impact and are reflected in the enhanced APN responsibilities of advocate, mentor, leader, educator, healthcare provider, and communicator. Most often people have a general idea about what values they think are personally important, yet a greater impact is found in stating the values that reflect who you are as a person.

The recognition of personal values is an essential step in the formation of professional identity because your values will form your behavior (Kidner 2019; Kinchen 2019; Samson 2009). Values of an APN can include compassion, competence, confidence, conscientious, commitment, and courage. The characteristics required for autonomous practice can include values of self-reliance, self-motivation, and high self-coping mechanisms (Vaismoradi et al. 2011). Therefore, self-perception and the embodiment of personal values directly impact the development of the APN professional identity.

The foundation of nursing is to provide holistic care that involves taking time to understand the wholeness of the person and to develop a healing partnership with the patient. This wellness paradigm is distinctly different than the medical model. APNs are in a unique position to design and promote care models that are patient-centered, and relationship-based with comprehensive systematic knowledge and skill that impact patients and communities (Kinchen 2019). This holistic care is built upon the values held true to nursing.

Personal values set the foundation on how you make decisions, organize your work life, and interact with friends, staff, students, family, and community. Personal and group beliefs and behavior are driven by the values upheld (Kinchen 2019). Values can provide direction and actions of groups and individuals (Purc and Laguna 2019). Many organizations have a set of written values. This section will focus on the recognition and incorporation of your personal values for your decision-making and actions.

6.5.2   What Are Values? Why Are Values Important?

These are great questions to ask. A simple way to understand values is that your values are the hidden drivers that push you to do what you believe is correct, your personal ethics, morals, motivation, and your behaviors.

6.5.3   Nursing Values and APN Nursing

Nursing values are the key components to several APN responsibilities including:

- APN as advocate
- APN as mentor
- APN as educator
- APN as formal leader
- APN as care provider
- APN as communicator
- APN as researcher
- APN as clinical expert
- APN as team leader
- APN as process and systems evaluator

Values often associated with nursing care include trust, integrity, kindness, caring, equity, and compassion.

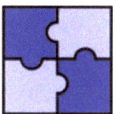

What values do you think are part of the APN role and responsibilities?
Example: To be an advocate, the values of trust and caring are essential.

APN Roles and Enhanced Responsibilities	Possible values
APN as advocate	
APN as mentor	
APN as educator	
APN as formal leader	
APN as care provider	
APN as communicator	
APN as researcher	
APN as clinical expert	
APN as team leader	
APN as process and systems evaluator	

What behaviors do you undertake as an APN student that reveal values that you feel are important?

Example: "I do not cheat on exams because I believe and portray the values honesty and integrity."

_____
_____
_____
_____
_____
_____
_____
_____

Common core nursing values in literature

- Human dignity
- Integrity
- Honesty
- Autonomy
- Altruism
- Social justice
- Privacy
- Precision and accuracy in caring
- Commitment
- Human relationship
- Sympathy
- Benevolence

- Individual and professional competency
- Professionalism
- Caring (Poorchangizi et al. 2019; Shahriari et al. 2013)

6.5.4   Nursing Values from a Graduate Student's Perspective

Although APN care is impacted by the values of the APN provider (you), those values are also influenced by the profession's ethical codes, and the social, economic, and religious conditions of the country (Poorchangizi et al. 2019). As values are internalized, they will become part of one's self-concept and professional identity. Research evaluating from a student's perspective concerning values in nursing revealed several values nursing students felt were important to provide high-quality and safe care (Poorchangizi et al. 2019):

6.5.5   Values from a Student's Perspective and Actions That Promote the Value

- Trust building and personal trust
  - Engage in on-going self-evaluation
  - Accept responsibility and accountability for own practice
  - Seek additional education to update knowledge and skills
  - Building strong relationships with all APN stakeholders
  - Improve communication, decrease passive aggression, and improve outcomes
  - Be an effective and committed team member and employee
  - Exemplify autonomous care through actions and documentation of your clinical practice
  - Complete the actions that you said you would complete
- Justice
  - Protect the health and safety of the public
  - Promote equitable access to nursing and healthcare
  - Meet the needs of a culturally diverse population
  - Persistence as patient advocacy
  - Promote team member equality
  - Uphold the ethical and moral standards of providing healthcare to all
- Professionalism
  - Participate in peer reviews
  - Evaluate and update standards of nursing care with evidence-based data
  - Initiate actions to improve environments of practice
  - Improve outcome measurements of high-quality care
  - Mentor, guide, and lead others
  - Act professional in all interactions
- Activism
  - Participate in policy concerning nursing and health
  - Participate in nursing research and implement findings
  - Maintain membership in a professional nursing organization

- – Be an advocate for the nursing profession
- – Actively educate the public on the nursing roles, education requirements, and impact
- – Promote all nurses working at their full scope of practice
- Caring
  - – Maintain patient confidentiality
  - – Safeguard patient's right to privacy
  - – Act as a patient advocate
  - – Respect each person as person first
  - – Listen to the patient's story and develop patient-centered care plan
  - – Provide same care with kindness to all people
  - – Do not engage in any form of lateral or vertical misconduct (Barlow et al. 2018; Poorchangizi et al. 2019)

Nursing students learn and incorporate the country's nursing values in their educational programs and through clinical rotations. This process could include a formal process to study and apply values in the workplace through ethical decisions-making discussion in post-clinical settings (Barlow et al. 2018). Your nursing experience has impacted your sense of values that are important to yourself, your work, your patients, your workplace, and the nursing profession.

6.5.6 Paying Attention to Values

Since values are essential components of your professional identity, it is wise to understand the research of values and implications of the values you chose. A significant contributor to the research on values was by the social psychologist, Milton Rokeach in 1973 with his publication "The Nature of Human Values." His work is still used today (Oceja et al. 2019).

There are two distinct types of personal values: Terminal and Instrumental.

Terminal values are the goals you want to achieve in your lifetime. These values signify the most important achievements in one's life (called end-states). Terminal values are the highest values in a person's value system and are motivational because they represent super goals beyond the immediate (Rokeach 1973). Terminal values are an expression of individual views of what is "moral" (Oceja et al. 2019).

Instrumental values are values used in our day-to-day lives. Generally, these values are anchors to guide your behavior. These values tend to be personal and intrapersonal focused and impact self-esteem and ways an individual would follow to achieve the aims in his life (Rokeach 1973). Instrumental values are motivating because they are instrumental in attaining one's end goals. These values can lead to conflicts since can they differ within a group (Tuulik et al. 2016).

Terminal and instrumental values represent two separate, yet functionally interconnected value systems. All of your chosen values impact modes of behavior and are instrumental to the attainment of all the values concerning end-states (Tuulik et al. 2016). Table 6.1 provides you with a list of terminal and instrumental values to help clarify and differentiate between the two types of values.

Table 6.1 Terminal and Instrumental values

Terminal values	Instrumental values
A world at peace (free of war and conflict)	Ambitious, broad-minded, capable, cheerful, courageous, helpful, and forgiving.
Family security (taking care of loved ones)	Cheerful (light-hearted, joyful)
Freedom (independence, free choice)	Love (affectionate, tender)
Equality (brotherhood, equal opportunity for all)	Honest (sincere, truthful)
Self-respect (self-esteem)	Self-control (restrained, self-discipline)
Happiness (contentedness)	Capable (competent, effective)
Wisdom (a mature understanding of life)	Ambitious (hard-working, aspiring)
National security (protection from attack)	Polite (courteous, well mannered)
True friendship (close companionship)	Imaginative (daring, creative)
Salvation (saved eternal life)	Independent (self-reliant, self-sufficient)
A sense of accomplishment (a lasting contribution)	Intellectual (intelligent, reflective)
A world of beauty (beauty of nature and the arts)	Broad-minded (open-minded)
A comfortable life (a prosperous life)	Logical (consistent, rational)
An exciting life (a stimulating active life)	Courageous (standing up for your beliefs)
Social recognition (respect, admiration)	Obedient (dutiful, respectful)
Mature love (sexual and spiritual intimacy)	Helpful (working for the welfare of others)
Inner harmony (freedom from inner conflict)	Responsible (dependable, reliable)
Pleasure (an enjoyable leisurely life)	Clean (neat, tidy)

6.5.7   Steps for Determining Values

Choosing your values can be difficult because there are so many values you may think are important to your nursing role. Within your personal transition plan, it is best to focus on only three or four values as your primary values of focus. These values should be reflected in everything you do. People should see those values in you every day from small to important tasks; from the activities you do with friends to those critical decisions you make professionally. These three to four values will serve as your foundation.

Step 1: Review Values
To know your values and have them clearly stated will set the foundation for you to empower and inspire others. Consider each of the values below in respect to yourself. This is not a complete list. You may have additional values that are important to you. This strategic plan is centered on your successful APN role transition. Therefore, the values should be instrumental values that refer to modes of behavior.

POTENTIAL PERSONAL VALUES (Instrumental values)

- Integrity
- Innovation
- Charity (time, talent, and treasure)
- Trust—Trustworthiness—Trust building
- Fortitude
- Honesty
- Quality
- Excellence
- Accountability
- Respect
- Communication
- Engaging or Engagement
- Altruism
- Leading change
- Service
- Commitment
- Team
- Professionalism
- Curiosity
- Collaboration
- Servitude
- Timeliness
- Kindness
- Consistency
- Adaptability
- Responsibility
- Dignity

- Creativity
- Adventurous
- Advocate
- Diligence
- Courage
- Ownership
- Clarity
- Diversity
- Knowledge
- Persevere or perseverance
- Wisdom
- Reflection
- Justice
- Caring
- Activism
- Gentleness
- Self-resiliency
- Equity
- Educator
- Freedom
- Humanity
- Generosity
- Endurance
- Success
- Balance
- Spirituality-Faith
- Forgiveness
- Respect

> What Strengths in your SWOT reflect a value? Write your strengths, then link your strengths to values

- _____
- _____
- _____

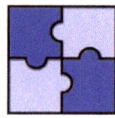

Circle the values that are important to you.

Step 2: Start Your Personal Value List

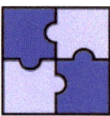

Choose five core values that reflect who you are and explain why the chosen value is meaningful to you:

1. _____
2. _____
3. _____
4. _____
5. _____

Step 3: Reveal and Reflect on Values

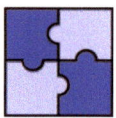

Choose a group of 2–3 people you know well. Ask them to write down or share what values they think YOU reflect. It is important to understand what values you are upholding daily without even knowing.

If you are completing this assignment with fellow students, or peers, in small groups tell each other what values each person reflects. What are the behaviors do you see in them naturally? Discuss thoughts on values.

Next, review the list of your chosen values and the values others say you reflect. Are some of the values the same? Now choose 3 (best) or 4 (the most) personal core values that you will uphold every day all the time.

Step 4: Write Your Final Personal Values List

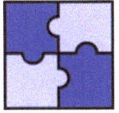

My core values are the values that I will uphold in my decisions, in my workplace, at home, in the community, and even in my quiet time alone. My chosen core values are:

1. _____
2. _____
3. _____
4. _____

What do personal values have to do with the role of the APN and APN responsibilities?
Personal values and values in a workplace set the behaviors that are acceptable. The role of the APN is to provide safe, high-quality healthcare to those in need. Therefore, the role of the APN demands integrity, accountability, innovation, and resiliency to name a few. Within the roles of APN as Leader, APN as Advocate, APN as mentor, APN as educator, APN as healthcare provider you can see how values will drive the expected behavior required to accomplish the role of the APN.

Thought Question: If you are an APN at a clinical setting that states integrity as a value. However, many of the staff arrive ½ to 1 h late for work every day without any concerns from the leadership.

Is integrity to work being upheld? _____. How you think allowing staff to arrive when they please will impact the workplace or patient care?

_____
_____
_____
_____
_____
_____

6.5.8   Values and Looking at Your Graduate Program or Workplace

Now that you understand that personal values are important and need to be reviewed daily. Review your graduate program, or workplace strategic plan. Are values listed? (Some organizations do not have stated values). This question is to help you understand that values drive behavior. Answer the question and then share in your group. Discuss the common values identified.

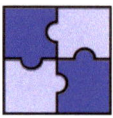

Write your workplace's (or university) stated values:

_____

1. Value _____ What actions or behaviors do you see? Give an example of good or bad example of an action, or behavior for that value.

_____
_____
_____

2. Value _____ What actions or behaviors do you see? Give an example of good or bad example of an action, or behavior for that value.

_____
_____
_____

3. Value _____ What actions or behaviors do you see? Give an example of good or bad example of an action, or behavior for that value.

_____
_____
_____

4. Value _____ What actions or behaviors do you see? Give an example of good or bad example of an action, or behavior for that value.

_____
_____
_____

6.6   Step 2 Building Your PTP: A Vision Statement

6.6.1   Background

The Vision is the "**WHAT**" to Accomplish

The foundation to personal success is **creating your personal VISION STATEMENT**. In your PTP, this vision statement is a short statement that says you will have a successful APN role transition. Although, you will soon learn that your PTP vision statement is not as simple as, "I will have a successful APN role transition!" There is a set process to developing a PTP vision statement, and this process starts with understanding the background thoughts that impact our future. In most people, these thoughts are in their subconscious because few people innately understand the importance of a strategic review of their future hopes and aspirations.

Most people have not taken the time to sit and think about what they want to be doing in 6 months, a year, or 3–5 years. If you wonder about the future, but never set a goal or plan, then it will be unlikely you will obtain your desired future. There is a process to develop your own vision. If you try, you will succeed, and developing a vision is the second step (after values) in putting direction into your professional career, clarifying your professional identity as an APN, and developing a personal transition plan.

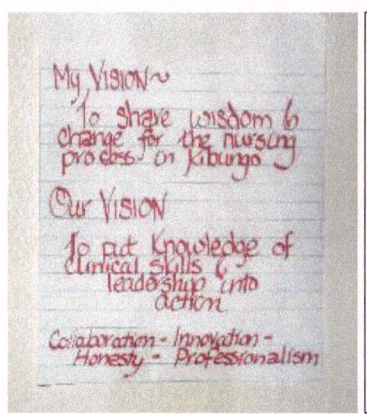

Example: When I was in Rwanda in 2014, this is what hung on my wall so I could look at it every day to make sure what I did that day and everyday- supported these Vision statements (One is mine, the other was the team I was working with). Every time I walked past my plan, I asked myself, "Did I uphold every value… every day" (bottom of paper). And "Did I strive towards the vision tatements… what did I do today that directly impacted our vision statement today?"

~ Maria Kidner DNP, FNP-BC, FAANP

6.6.2   Step for Creating a Vision Statement

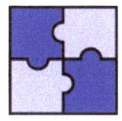

Step 1: Review your gifts, passions, and short-term and long-term APN role transition desires. Write down some of your ideas, or concerns about your APN role transition.

Notes:_____
_____
_____
_____

Step 2: Determine the true essence of why you want to become an APN

> **A root cause analysis** is a process used to find the origin of a problem to determine what event/mistake happened and to discover possible reasons the mistake happened. Subsequently creative solutions can be evaluated and implemented to decrease the chance of the mistake from happening again. A root cause analysis allows for a unique structured process for an in-depth but narrow view of a potential cause. One type of root analysis is to ask the question "Why did this mistake happen?" and then ask why to the answer five times (Peerally et al. 2017; Toyoda 2020).

Using the technique of a root cause analysis of asking why you want to achieve your future desire, or goals, and taking that answer and asking why, then that answer and asking why…. asking for five (5) times allows you to get to the true essence of your desires. Often our unconscious thoughts can hide the true essence to the desire or complex goal. This introspection activity of asking why can be powerful in finding the real meaning behind a desire to achieve a specific goal or personal achievement.

In building a PTP, the process of a root analysis is used to determine the precise reason why you have chosen to become an APN and your anticipated future. The root analysis process applied to a vision statement development will help you to see your importance, strengths, hidden agendas, or expose barriers.

Review your desires you wrote for 3, 6, 12, and 24 months. Choose the desire that applies to you being a successful APN. You can also answer the question, "I want to become an APN because…."

This is called a "passion statement."

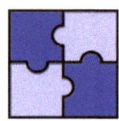

Write your personal passion statement concerning your APN role transition:

"I want to…_____"

There are TWO ways to evaluate the true essence of your desired APN role: (1) Why is this important? Or (2) What is the barrier preventing me to obtain my aspired achievement target? Below is a vision root analysis table. It is recommended that you read this entire section and consider the examples before working on your PTP vision build process. Step 2 and Step 3 are closely related and are shown together in the examples.

Step 2. Complete the Vision Root Analysis

Why do you want to become an APN? What do you aspire to accomplish when you are an APN?	What do I feel is a barrier/fear to becoming a successful APN?
#1 Why is the above response important?	#1 Why is the above response important?
#2 Why is the above response important?	#2 Why is the above response important?
#3 Why is the above response important?	#3 Why is the above response important?
#4 Why is the above response important?	#4 Why is the above response important?
#5 Why is the above response important?	#5 Why is the above response important?

Step 3: Making options.

In a root analysis, the fourth and fifth answers tend to provide an insight into the true desires, or reasons, someone would like to accomplish the initial stated aspiration, or desire for personal achievement (APN role transition, or APN accomplishment). Using a triangle as a graphic is helpful in recognizing options of the vision.

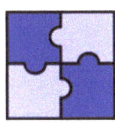

Build your Triangle. *After reviewing the examples,* build a triangle with your aspiration for a successful APN role transition and place Why # 4 and Why #5 on your triangle

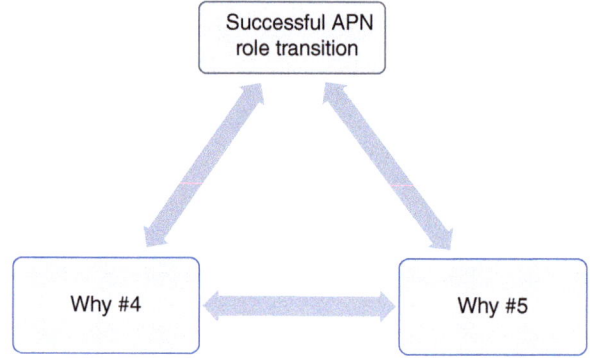

Olivier's Example: "*I want to become an APN so I can empower nurses to be their best.*"

Root cause analysis	Olivier's answers
#1 Why do you want to become an APN? *"I want to become an APN so I can empower nurses to be their best."*	*"Because nurses can improve the health of people and communities."*
#2 Why is it important that nurses help other?	*"Because when people (nurses and patients) have knowledge about being healthier, then they can find ways to become healthier."*
#3 Why is becoming healthier important?	*"Because healthier people have more happiness and kindness."*
#4 Why is the having more happiness and kindness important?	*"Because people would have the ability to do more opportunities in life."*
#5 Why is achieving opportunities important?	*"Because healthy people can be creative for the good of the community."*

```
        ┌─────────────────┐
        │  Be a successful │
        │       APN        │
        └─────────────────┘
          ↗              ↘
┌──────────────┐      ┌──────────────┐
│    More      │ ←──→ │ Good of the  │
│ oppurtunities│      │  community   │
└──────────────┘      └──────────────┘
```

Judy's Example of a BARRIER

   "*I am afraid to enter the APN role because I fear being bullied or nurses treating me poorly due to jealousy.*"

Root cause analysis	Judy's answers
Why are you afraid of your pending APN role transition?	*Because I am afraid of being bullied or nurses treating me poorly due to jealousy*
Why 1—Why are you afraid of vertical/lateral workplace violence?	*Because I do not handle conflict well*
Why 2—Why do you not handle conflict well?	*Because I feel vulnerable … yet I have the capacity to achieve my vision of APN*
Why 3—Why do you feel vulnerable?	*Because I lack the skills to see and overcome passive aggression*
Why 4—What do you lack?	*I lack knowledge on how to develop strong trust relationships and courage against workplace violence*
Why 5—What do trust relationships have to do with violence and your APN role?	*Trust is built upon justice, respect, and integrity of all providing healthcare. As a team we are successful.*

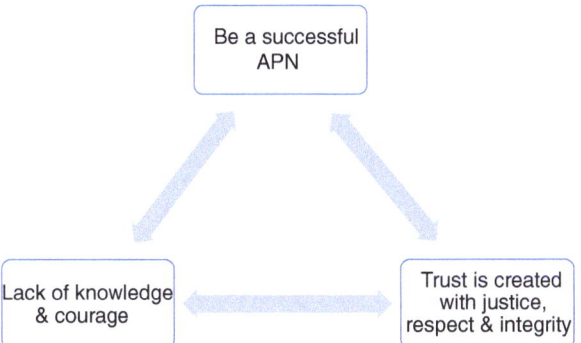

Now return to the blank root analysis and vision build triangle and complete your working vision build sheet. You may want to try a few different passion statements to find the root analysis that really connects with you about your personal progress of APN role transition.

Step 4: Decide your action that is required to achieve the "Why #4 and 5"

You need TO DO something to achieve your successful APN role transition. What is the action you need to complete your personal aspiration? This process creates motion. What is the action you need to complete your desire for personal advancement?

- To have
- To mentor
- To inspire
- To exemplify
- To promote
- To influence
- To guide
- To immerse
- To build
- To accept
- To experience

- To embody
- To behold
- To explore
- To cultivate
- To attain
- To discover
- To distinguish
- To gain
- To accomplish
- To develop
- To recognize

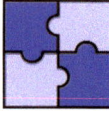

Can you think of other actions?

_____

_____

_____

Circle the action you want to use to assist your role transition. Choose 5–8 actions you think you will need to do to accomplish a successful role transition. Having choices of actions can help you be creative in the wording of your vision and mission statements.

Step 5: Consider and choose your action(s) and determine your triangle fit.

This step provides you with three or four different statements using different arrangements of actions. This step is like moving the three components of your triangle into different sequence until you find the fit. Use different actions to help find the perfect fit of words. Review the following examples before completing step 5 with your personal transition plan.

6.6.3   Vision Build Example for Actions

Example 1: Olivier's Personal Role Transition Plan

"I want to become an APN so I can empower nurses to be their best."

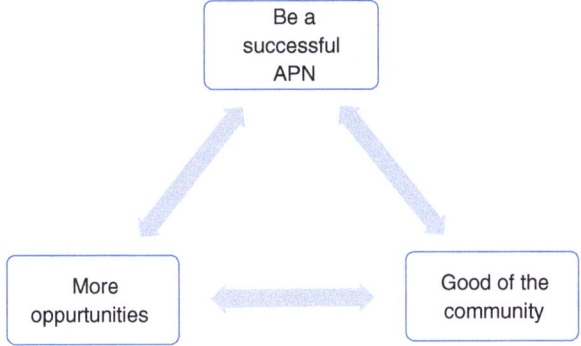

- **Actions:** to educate, to share, to empower, to embody, to cultivate, to inspire, to improve, to attain, to mentor
- **Mix and Match: For my successful APN role transition I will…**
- inspire and cultivate knowledge to patients and staff to increase health, happiness, and creativity as a successful APN.
- share knowledge and empower others to obtain healthy habits for life, creativity, and happiness as a successful APN.
- impact patients, peers, and community through shared wisdom on health, illness, and life to improve the happiness and opportunities of all as a successful APN.

Example 2
Judy's Personal Transition Plan: *"I am afraid to enter the APN role because I fear being bullied or nurses treating me poorly due to jealousy."*

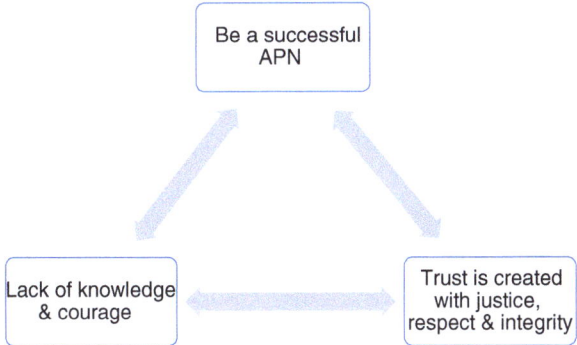

- **Actions:** to build, to support, to promote, to attain, to gain, to communicate, to experience
- **Mix and Match: As a successful APN I will…**
- gain knowledge and communication skills to build trust relationships based on respect and justice to have a successful APN role transition and decrease nursing role transition bulling.
- experience success as APN through the development of excellent communication skills to build trust relationships with all involved with my patients.
- support respect, justice, and integrity through gained skills in trust relationship building for APN role transition success.

Example 3
In this example the student had a specific desire to achieve to obtain a sense of success. This is another way to consider the reason why you personally desire to become an APN.

William's Personal Transition plan   *"I want to become an APN to be an expert in pharmacokinetics."*

Personal aspiration	I want to become an APN to be an expert in pharmacokinetics
Why 1	Because I lack experience with many medications
Why 2	Because medications treat diseases and health problems
Why 3	Because good treatment can improve the health and wellness of patients
Why 4	Because they can have a better quality of life (QOF)
Why 5	To increase happiness of my patients

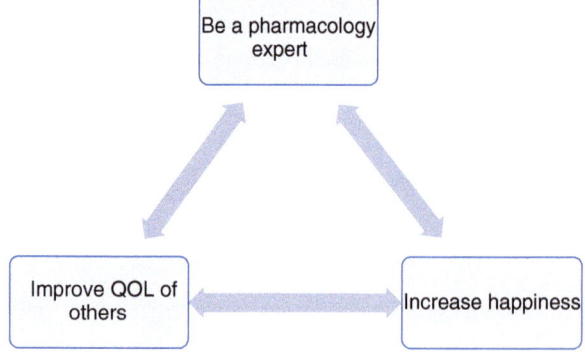

Actions to help, to become, to improve, to attain, to mentor, to exemplify, to promote, to influence, to increase

Mix and Match
- I will become an expert in pharmacology as APN to help improve the QOL of others and thus increase their happiness.
- I will use pharmacology expertly as APN to help others increase their happiness through an improved quality of life.
- As an APN, I will maximize correct pharmacology to improve quality of life of my patients.
- I will help others gain happiness through improved QOL from personalized and effective pharmacology.

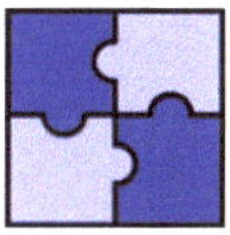

Your turn: Use your passion statement for your role transition root analysis, set your triangle, determine your desired actions, and then mix and match for a potential vision statement.

I want to be an APN because:

_____

Or

I am afraid of my APN role transition because:

_____

Your APN personal transition plan root analysis

Root analysis of why you want to become an APN	Answer
#1 Why?	
#2 Why?	
#3 Why?	
#4 Why?	
#5 Why?	

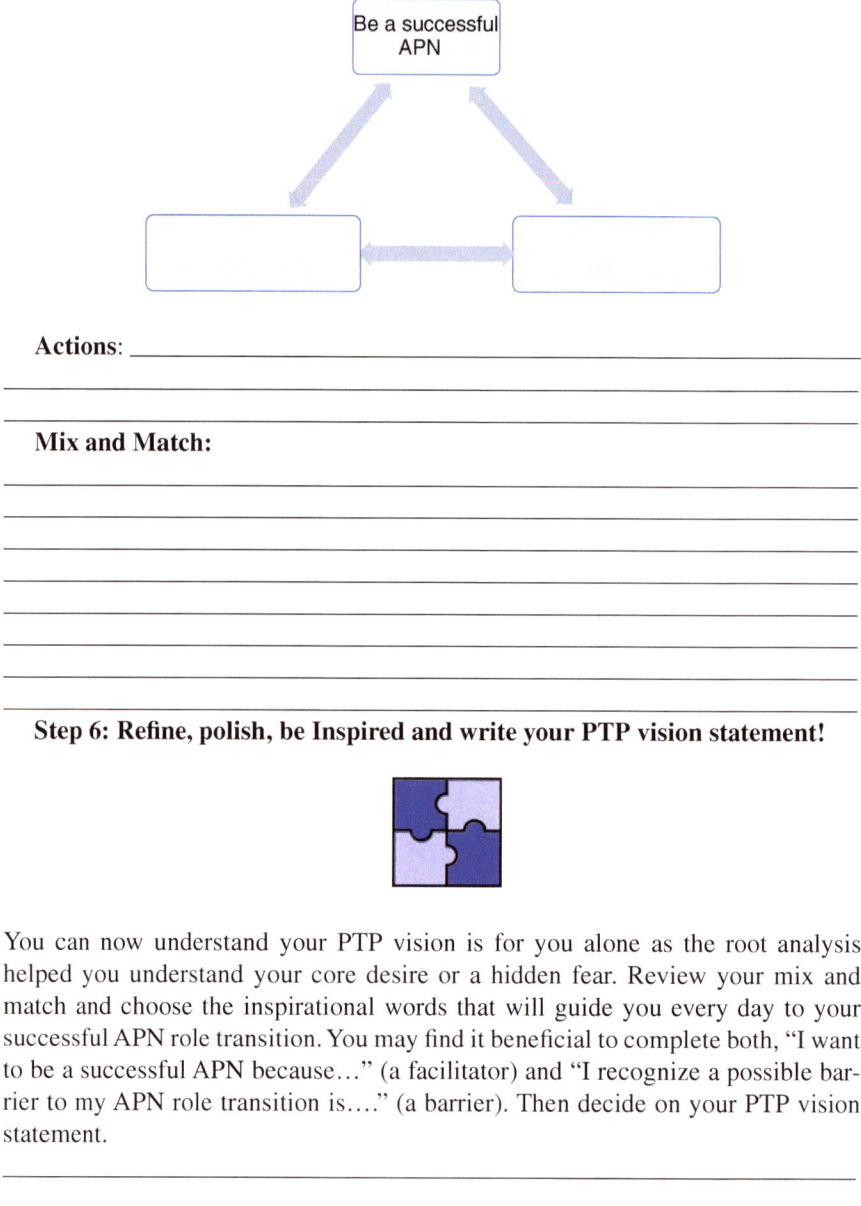

Actions: _____

_____

Mix and Match:

_____
_____
_____
_____
_____
_____
_____

Step 6: Refine, polish, be Inspired and write your PTP vision statement!

You can now understand your PTP vision is for you alone as the root analysis helped you understand your core desire or a hidden fear. Review your mix and match and choose the inspirational words that will guide you every day to your successful APN role transition. You may find it beneficial to complete both, "I want to be a successful APN because…" (a facilitator) and "I recognize a possible barrier to my APN role transition is…." (a barrier). Then decide on your PTP vision statement.

_____
_____
_____
_____

6.6.4   My Personal Transition Plan Vision Statement

_____

_____

Step 7: Post your vision statement.

What good is your vision statement if you hide it in this book and never say your vision statement to yourself and other? Write you vision statement and place it where you can see it every day.

6.7   Step 3: Building Your PTP—Developing a Mission Statement

Once you have your PTP set in a vision statement, you will need to determine how you want to accomplish your successful APN role transition and to whom it will impact. That is your mission.

> **The Mission Statement is the HOW to accomplish the VISION & WHOM you will impact**

Mission statement background

The mission defines how your vision will be accomplished. The mission also identifies your stakeholders (the whom your vision will impact) and acknowledges what your stakeholders want. Your mission statement should give you a process of how you will achieve your vision statement.

Mission statements are important to APN PTP

- For APN role transition and professional identity growth, the mission statement can provide the process to achieve successful role transition.
- For your professional identity growth, the mission statement can provide the process to achieve successful role transition.

6.7.1   Your Mission Statement Build Guide

Step 1: Determine whom you, as APN will affect. These people are called "stakeholders." "Stakeholders" are people who are impacted by you and your vision. Who are your stakeholders?

Personal Stakeholders

For a personal mission statement, your stakeholders could include family, friends, and colleagues. Or your stakeholder could be implied as everybody. For example, in the vision statement: *"As APN I will inspire curiosity and mentor courage and help others surpass possibilities,"* the *"help others"* means anybody and everybody.

Possible stakeholders for personal and personal professional vision statements

- Self
- Family
- Colleagues
- Staff/team
- Physicians
- Patients and their families
- The workplace/organization
- The formal senior leadership
- The professional organization
- The body that writes the laws about your scope and role
- The local community
- Instructors and/or preceptors
- Mentors
- Nurses: generalist, specialty care, and APN

Example of Stakeholders and Impact

Lori Carlson is a new APN joining a clinic that provides care to the homeless. Her vision statement, "With dignity and respect for all, as APN I will help save lives of our patients."

Lori has identified her stakeholders, and stated her desired impact on each:

- *Zereck, the **social worker**—*to integrate behavior health and physical health into one platform
- *Trish, the **case manager**—*to encourage her through her master's degree program and inspire curiosity into integrative care
- *Becky, the **medical assistant*** (an aid to nursing)—to build ownership and engagement through increased responsibilities in the laboratory
- *Thomas the **client liaison/appointments/triage**—*to create collaborative partnerships with patients, team, and community
- *The **company's senior leadership team**—*to show the improved outcomes with an integrated team working on the same goals
- *The **Board of directors**—*to gain commitment through trust relationships built on integrity
- *The **local emergency response groups**—*to build collaborative relationships
- *The **homeless/patients**—*to inspire to be an active participant in becoming healthier

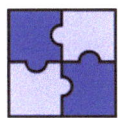

Who are your stakeholders for your stated PTP Vision statement?

_____
_____
_____
_____

Step 2: The mission is a statement of how you will obtain your vision and to whom. This step is to identify your "who" or the people who will be impacted by your vision and determine what actions you would like to accomplish to each stakeholder. Review the example of stakeholders and impact with APN Lori, then fill out your table of stakeholders.

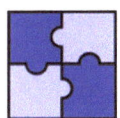

List your stakeholder. Identify what you want "to do" for each stakeholder, or how do you want to impact each group/or person. These are "to do _____" statements. To understand the importance of your actions, you can clarify your thoughts by answering why that impact is important for that stakeholder.

Stakeholder (WHO)	Wanted impact and why important	HOW to achieve impact (action)

Step 2: In this step you need to determine how you are going to accomplish your vision.

- **Example of Lori**—Why do you want to become a successful APN?
- *Vision: With dignity and respect for all, as APN I will help save our patients.*
- How do you want to accomplish your vision?
- *"I want to build an engaged integrative care team based on our values of integrity, innovation, and communication. I want to train to save lives."*

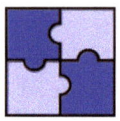

How do you want to accomplish your vision?

_____
_____
_____
_____
_____

Step 4: This step is to clarify the action(s) you will need to successfully achieve your vision (your APN role transition). Review your actions from the stakeholders list and determine the main actions you want to do to

Example of Lori— *"The action I want to create is to collaborate, to cultivate, to express, to explore, to surpass, to build, to encourage, and to integrate."*

Review your stakeholders and choose your actions:

_____
_____
_____

Step 5: Tie your Vision (the What) to the activity in your Mission (the How) with your values (the why)

Review the vision examples before writing your own. The process of developing your PTP can take time and several rewrites until you are satisfied the words that share what your heart intended. Do not worry if what you have written is not perfect. The precise words will come. The important part is to write your values, vision, and mission and post them on your wall. As you walk by and review your daily progress, the perfect words will form… then you can modify and perfect your APN personal transition plan.

Your values should be identified in your mission statement because your values drive your behaviors. It is through your actions you will achieve your vision.

Example of Lori—NOTE: This Example Is from Lori's Personal Workplace Strategic Plan
Values: *integrity, innovation, and communication*
   Vision: *With dignity and respect for all, as APN I will help save our patients*
   Actions: *to show, to gain, to develop, to build, to create, to implement, to integrate, to encourage, to inspire.*
   Mission: *Working together as a team with **integrity**, we will develop, implement, and expand a whole health integrated team that support the gaining of knowledge, respect, and trust of all involved through **innovative** healthcare delivery, a dedication to learning, and open **communications**.*

Note: Lori's values are embedded in her mission statement (bolded). Plus, Lori's stated "team" are all of her stakeholders listed. The use of team with the inclusion of her patients, board of directors, and the emergency response team will require specific goals and action plans to ensure inclusion and a fully integrated healthcare model.

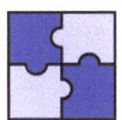

Your APN role transition Mission Build Steps
List your Values: _____
Complete the table.

Mission build steps	Your answers
1. Determine your stakeholders	
2. State what you want to accomplish with your mission?	
3. State your stakeholders and the desired impact on each stakeholder	Review your table you created
4. What action(s) do you want to create to achieve?	Obtain from steps 2 and 3
5. Tie your vision (the what) to the activity in your mission (the how) with your values (the why).	

Mission build steps	Your answers
6. Refine and write your mission statement to provide the "how" you will accomplish your vision and "to whom" your vision statement will impact. You may have two sentences (if needed).	See below

Step 6. This last step combines all of the aspects of the mission: the how you will accomplish your vision, identifies your stakeholders, and finally ties your values to your mission statement.

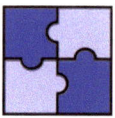

Review ideas for your mission statement to provide the "how" you will accomplish your vision and "to whom" your vision statement will impact. Refine and complete your mission statement on how you will work towards your successful APN role transition.

My Mission Statement. **Note: Your Mission Statement can be 1–2 sentences.**

_____
_____
_____
_____
_____

6.8   Step 4 Building Your PTP: Goals

Goals are your big steps required to implement your mission statement. Goals are easy to determine if you have well-written vision and mission statements. Your PTP goals are the big steps you need to accomplish for your successful APN role transition. Review the following examples before completing your own goals.

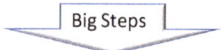

6.8.1   Goals Examples

Example 1: Olivier's PTP
Values commitment, knowledge, creativity

Mission *I will have a successful APN role transition through my* **commitment** *to share knowledge with staff, patients, and community. I will empower others to use* **knowledge** *to positively impact life, happiness, and* **creativity** *within my community.*

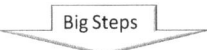

1. Gain knowledge on pathophysiology, pharmacology, and lifestyle management
2. Develop educational activities for peers, staff, patients, and community on specific topics
3. Implement educational activities
4. Seek follow-up or outcome measurements to ensure I have educated and impacted others

Example 2: Judy's PTP
Values   perseverance, communication, trust relationships

Mission *I will have a successful APN role transition through my dedication and* **perseverance** *to effective* **communication** *and* **trust relationships***. I will seek to understand, build my communication skills to decrease vertical and lateral workplace bullying, and mentor integrity.*

1. Study and practice techniques to build trust relationships
2. Obtain knowledge and skills to recognize and address workplace passive aggressive behaviors
3. Practice communication skills to develop courage and confidence to respond in a professional and positive manner when confronted with passive aggression
4. Seek and obtain a mentor through the role transition process

Example 3: William's PTP
Values   *communication, knowledge, commitment*

Mission *I will have a successful APN role transition through my* **commitment** *to* **knowledge** *gain of pharmacology so I can improve the QOL of others with excellent* **communication** *and shared decision makers and my prescription plans.*

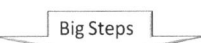

1. Work hard to gain pharmacology knowledge
2. Develop excellent communication
3. Develop processes for shared decision-making

Example 4: Lori's PTP

Values *integrity, innovation, and communication*

Mission *I will have a successful APN role transition when I can implement processes where working together as a team, we will develop, implement, and expand a whole health integrated team that support the gaining of knowledge, respect, and trust of all involved through innovative healthcare delivery, a dedication to learning, and open communications.*

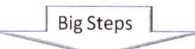

1. Gain knowledge and skills in team building and management
2. Understand and develop personal clinical leadership style
3. Use knowledge sharing as a means to build trust relationship
4. Review current and possible healthcare delivery systems, seek innovation for new processes
5. Work on the team workplace culture concerning respect and open communications

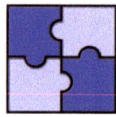

STEP 1: Review your mission statement and determine the big steps to accomplish your mission. You may only have 1–2 needed big steps, or your mission may be more complex and require more goals.

1. _____
2. _____
3. _____
4. _____
5. _____

6.9   Step 5: Building Your PTP—Action Plans

The fifth step in your PTP is to determine the action needed to accomplish your big steps.

6.9.1   Action Plans Background

The tasks you need to achieve to accomplish your goal are called "Action Plans." The important part of creating action plans is detail. If you have great goal and only vague action plans, you may not succeed.

Rationale for Detailed Action Plans

If your goal is, *"I will graduate with my master's degree."* Next you write an action plan of: *"I will need to study."* You might not become successful because life is complex and too many other activities demand time and attention. However, if you devise a specific action plan and stick to that plan, then you created a plan to develop excellent study habits. The effective, detailed action plan would be: *"I will study at the library for 3 h on Tuesdays and Thursdays and 6 h on Saturday."*

You want your vision statement to be phenomenally successful, therefore you need properly constructed, detailed action plans that will provide a clear path to achieve your vision (Ogbeiwi 2017). To create a detailed action plan is to make sure each statement is "SMART." This basic framework provides a logical structure to provide clear directions for actions (Ogbeiwi 2017).

6.9.2   Action Plans Need To Be "SMART"

- **S = Specific**. Be precise about what you want to accomplish. What is the specific outcome?
- **M = Measurable**. State a measurable indicator of the desired outcome.
- **A = Attainable**. You must have an opportunity (either have or can obtain the skills, knowledge, equipment, and time) to achieve the needed tasks. Plus, you need to state an achievable relevant target of the above indicator.
- **R = Realistic**. The target level can be attained with your current skills, knowledge, finances, and abilities within a reasonable time frame.
- **T = Time**. Each action/task must have a time component and a completion date specified (Ogbeiwi 2017)

Example   *Fausta's Strategic Plan.*

Fausta is an APN associate professor for her University's School of Nursing. She reported a frustration on the death rate of newborns in the newborn intensive care unit.

Her #5 of the "whys" root cause analysis: Why is there high mortality and morbidity rate of newborns? "Because lack of knowledge taught and no mentors to make habits."

WHY   Values: * **Integrity** * **Quality** * **Collaboration** * **Advocacy**

WHAT Vision Statement: *"To save newborn lives through sharing of **knowledge and advocacy**."*

HOW Mission Statement: *"Driven by **integrity**; I will become a qualified neonatal nurse at the **doctorate level** and **advocate** at international and national levels through a **collaborative** network with neonatal working groups for **quality** care. I will conduct research and healthcare professional mentorship in order to help nurses and midwives to develop their competencies in neonatal care to save newborn lives."*

The identified Big Steps—Goals
1. *Get accepted into a PhD program*
2. ***Find opportunities to be an advocate on the national and international levels***
3. *Conduct research in neonatology*
4. *Become a mentor*

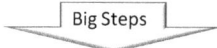

6.9.3   Fausta's Big Step #2

Fausta determined she needed to discuss this goal with her mentor. In the discussion it was determined that the Dean of the School of Nursing assigned the people to conferences when opportunities arose.

Thus, her SMART Action Plans were:
1. ***I will*** *call the Dean's office within the next 2 days and make an appointment with the Dean within the next 4 weeks.*
2. ***I will*** *bring a written copy of my Personal Strategic Plan to give to the Dean at the meeting and discuss my Strategic Plan with special emphasis on goal #2.*
3. ***I will*** *write down 5 talking points and practice my presentation to the Dean 3 times for 3 days to prepare.*
4. ***I will*** *write a Thank you note to the Dean for her time and consideration and deliver the note within 48 h of the meeting.*
5. *When I receive an opportunity to be an advocate on the national or international level, **I will** create a new short-term strategic plan within the first week to ensure my success.*

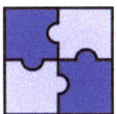

Review Fausta's specific action plans. Are they SMART? Why or why not?

_____

_____

_____

Outcome Fausta was given the responsibility to design and implement an international conference for saving newborns. At the previous conference there were 34 attendees. The conference she implemented hosted over 300 nurses, physicians, and health workers from multiple countries. She won the 2019 Council of International Neonatal Nurses Award for her leadership and passion. She started her PhD education in 2020 and is eager to be part of the full engagement of the APN role in Rwanda.

6.9.4   Your SMART Action Plan Build Guide

STEP 1: SMART Action Plans:

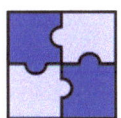

Think of 3–5 specific steps that need to be accomplished under each big step (Goal). Each step needs to be Specific-Measurable-Attainable-Realistic- and Time bound. Completing this process will help your role transition by creating a great plan for graduate education, clinicals, home life, and other responsibilities, thereby helping to decrease the stress, anxiety, and uncertainty often associated with APN role transition. In addition, when you develop SMART Action Plans you are forced to look to the future and the possibility of obtaining your vision! You can obtain your vision. This process of designing, writing, and posting your personal transition plan will help you understand yourself and yourself as nurse, as APN, as a healthcare provider, and as an APN leader. You can be highly successful in your APN role transition.

Write your ideas of what you need to achieve your goals for your personal role transition plan.

_____

_____

_____

STEP 2: "I will…" statements.

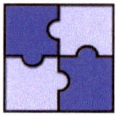

Write each Action Plan in the positive and strong voice starting with, "I will…" These "I will" statements are the specific actions you will do to achieve your goals and written in a SMART fashion.

1. I will _____
   Specific outcome desired—(who, what, when, how):
   _____
   _____
   Measurable—how will you know you have achieved this action plan?
   _____
   Attainable—do you have the skills, time, and knowledge to complete this action?
   Yes/ No Explain what skills/time/knowledge are needed:_____
   Realistic—Is this action plan realistic? Yes/No
   Time—be specific: _____

2. I will _____
   Specific outcome desired—(who, what, when, how):
   _____
   _____
   Measurable—how will you know you have achieved this action plan? _____
   _____
   Attainable—do you have the skills, time, and knowledge to complete this action?
   Yes/ No Explain what skills/time/knowledge are needed:_____
   Realistic—Is this action plan realistic? Yes/No
   Time—be specific: _____

3. I will _____
   Specific outcome desired—(who, what, when, how):
   _____
   _____
   Measurable—how will you know you have achieved this action plan? _____
   _____
   Attainable—do you have the skills, time, and knowledge to complete this action?
   Yes/ No Explain what skills/time/knowledge are needed: _____
   Realistic—Is this action plan realistic? Yes/No
   Time—be specific: _____

4. I will _____
   Specific outcome desired—(who, what, when, how):
   _____
   _____

Measurable—how will you know you have achieved this action plan? _____
_____

Attainable—do you have the skills, time, and knowledge to complete this action?
Yes/ No Explain what skills/time/knowledge are needed:_____
Realistic—Is this action plan realistic? Yes/No
Time—be specific: _____
5. I will _____
Specific outcome desired—(who, what, when, how):

_____
_____

Measurable—how will you know you have achieved this action plan? _____
_____

Attainable—do you have the skills, time, and knowledge to complete this action?
Yes/ No Explain what skills/time/knowledge are needed:_____
Realistic—Is this action plan realistic? Yes/No
Time—be specific: _____

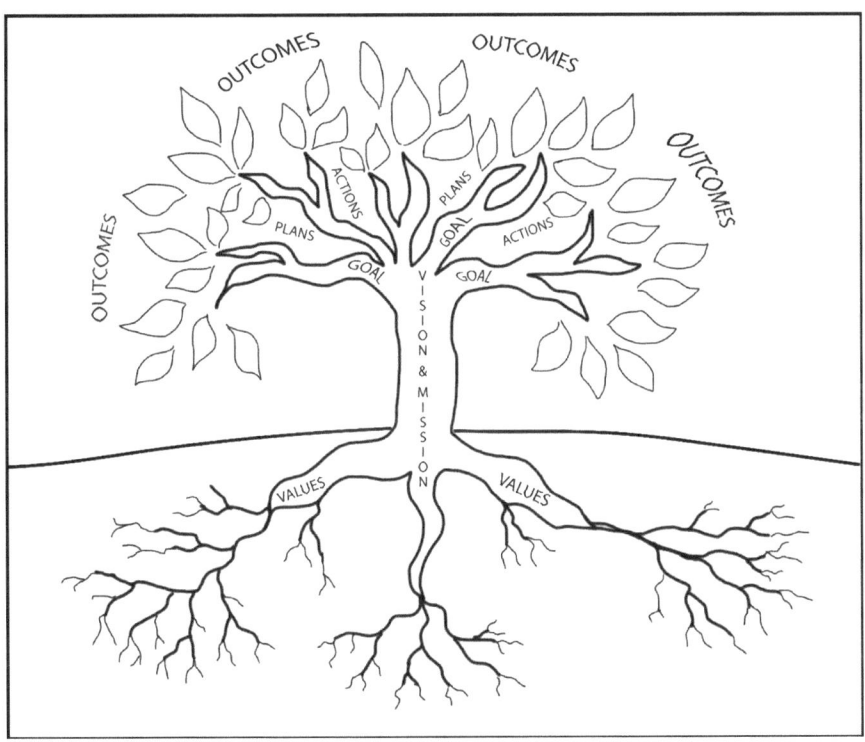

Fig. 6.1 Schematic drawing for a graphic model for strategic planning (Kidner 2019)

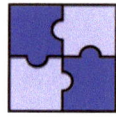

Now review your Mission statement and goals. Choose one goal and write at least two SMART Action Plans.

Goal: _____

Action Plan:

I will _____

_____

I will_____

_____

I will _____

_____

Congratulations! You have finished a complex process of building a PTP. Most people do not have a strategic plan because they have never seen a plan used daily to drive high quality and impactful outcomes. Although you built a PTP, the same process is used to strategically think and design processes for clinical projects, educational activities, teams, committees, or workplaces. The more you work with your PTP, the more comfortable you will become with building, implementing, and evaluating the success of strategic plans throughout your APN career. Figure 6.1 provides you a graphic representation of your PTP.

Think of your PTP as a huge, healthy tree. The roots tap deep into the soil where you find knowledge, skills, mentors, and support. The roots are your values (your WHY) that determine your behavior and what you hold true. Without strong values, you will not have a strong tree. The tree trunk is your Vision (your WHAT) and your Mission (your HOW). The branches are the big steps coming from your Vision and Mission—these branches are your Goals (the Big Steps). The leaves are your action plans (your "I will..."). The outcomes are the entire healthy, strong tree that requires all aspects to be whole and strong.

Complete your PTP and then post it on your wall so you can monitor your progress of your APN role transition.

6.9.5   Common Barriers to Action Plans

If you write an excellent plan, but do not implement your action plans, then you will not have a structured process for APN role transition.

Workplace Factors Barriers

1. Role ambiguity—If there is no clarity of the APN role in the workplace that reflects and supports the country's APN scope of practice, then it is difficult to smoothly role transition. As APN, you can make a difference by knowing what the workplace APN scope of practice and description. You can provide APN facts and help shape the understanding and trust of the APN role expand.

2. Vertical bullying and lateral bullying are detrimental to role transition, especially if the formal leadership is not part of the solution and supporting a healthy workplace culture.
3. Unequal distribution of resources. If resources are withheld from APNs, then it is difficult to provide the potential of APN care.

Personal Factors Barriers
1. Lack of introspective and self-exploration
2. Poor work–life balance
3. Low personal motivation
4. Poor personal coping mechanisms
5. Low self-resiliency
6. Poor self-concept
7. Poor self-efficacy
8. Low attachment to APN role; low professional identity

As you read this book, you can see common barriers and common facilitators to the success of APN role transition. It is important to remember that your role transition is personal to you. You are in control of your knowledge, skills, and personal development. You PTP is your personal map and guide to success. It is your choice to complete a PTP, and your choice to implement.

My Personal Strategic Plan

My Values: _____

My Vision: _____
_____

My Mission: _____
_____
_____
_____
_____

My Goal (My Big Step) #1
_____

My Action Plans. "I will…"
A. SMART: _____
_____

B. SMART: _____
_____

C. SMART: _____
_____

D. SMART: _____
_____

My Goal (My Big Step) #2

My Action Plans. "I will…"

A. SMART: _____

B. SMART: _____

C. SMART: _____

My Goal (My Big Step) #3

My Action Plans. "I will…"
A. SMART: _____

B. SMART: _____

C. SMART: _____

D. SMART:_____

My Goal (My Big Step) #4

My Action Plans. "I will…"
A. SMART: _____

B. SMART: _____

C. SMART: _____

D. SMART: _____

My Goal (My Big Step) #5

My Action Plans. "I will…"
A. SMART: _____

B. SMART: _____

C. SMART: _____

D. SMART: _____

6.10 Summary

This chapter is devoted to understanding and obtaining the skills to develop a personalized transition plan (PTP) for your APN role transition. Developing a PTP is important to the success of APN role transition as it will provide you a personal map and steps to obtain the APN role based upon an identified facilitator (something that inspired you to become and APN) or a barrier that may hinder your APN role transition. To develop a strong PTP you will need to recognize your passions, gifts, strengths, weaknesses, opportunities, and threats. Building a PTP develops the foundation of your professional identity through the self-reflections and setting of aspirations to achieve after in an APN clinical practice. The step-by-step process for you to develop your personal strategic plan is presented and includes:

- Values = **why** something is done
- Vision = **what** you want to accomplish
- Mission = **how** you are going to accomplish your "what" and "to whom"
- Goals = the **"Big Steps"** needed to achieve your vision and mission
- Action Plans = SMART **"I will"** statements that will provide specific directions to achieve each goal. These are your **"when"** plans.
  - Specific outcome
  - Measurable (a tool/way to measure the desired outcome)
  - Attainable (you have, or can obtain, the skill, knowledge, or tools)
  - Realistic
  - Time Bound

References

Bandura A (2018) Toward a psychology of human agency: pathways and reflections. Perspect Psychol Sci 13(2):130–136. https://doi.org/10.1177/1745691617699280

Barlow NA, Hargreaves J, Gillibrand W (2018) Nurses' contributions to the resolution of ethical dilemmas in practice. Nurs Ethics 25(2):230–242. https://doi.org/10.1177/0969733017703700

Barnes H (2015) Nurse practitioner role transition: a concept analysis. Nurs Forum 50(3): 137–146

Bryson JM, Edwards LH, Van Slyke DM (2018) Getting strategic about strategic planning research. Public Manag Rev 20(3):17–339. https://doi.org/10.1080/14719037.2017.1285111

Garcia EV (2016) Strategic planning: a tool for personal and career growth. Heart Asia 8:36–39. https://doi.org/10.1136/heartasia-2015-010684

Gibb's Reflective Cycle (n.d.). https://www.ed.ac.uk/reflection/reflectors-toolkit/reflecting-on-experience/gibbs-reflective-cycle. Accessed 17 Jul 2020

Higginbotham E, Church K (2012) Strategic planning as a tool for achieving alignment in academic health centers. Trans Am Clin Clim Assoc 123:292–303

Kidner M (2019) APN role transition with LEAP leadership. Copyright of unpublished works. TXu 2-166-138. The United States Copyright Office

Kinchen E (2019) Holistic nursing values in nurse practitioner education. Int J Nurs Educ Scholarsh 16(1):20180082

Markman KD, McMullen MN (2003) A reflection and evaluation model of comparative thinking. Personal Soc Psychol Rev 7(3):244–267. https://doi.org/10.1207/S15327957PTPR0703_04

Murphy M (2018) Neuroscience explains why you need to write down your goals if you actually want to achieve them. https://www.forbes.com/sites/markmurphy/2018/04/15/neuroscience-explains-why-you-need-to-write-down-your-goals-if-you-actually-want-to-achieve-them/#7cab23e27905. Accessed 23 Nov 2019

Oceja et al (2019) Revisiting the difference between instrumental and terminal values to predict (stimulating) prosocial behaviors: the transcendental-change profile. Br J Soc Psychol 58:749–768

Ogbeiwi O (2017) Why written objectives need to be SMART. Br J Healthcare Manag 23(7):324–336. https://doi.org/10.12968/bjhc.2017.23.7.324

Peerally MF, Carr S, Waring J et al (2017) The problem with root cause analysis. BMJ Qual Saf 26:417–422. https://doi.org/10.1136/bmjqs-2016-005511

Poorchangizi B, Borhani F, Abbsazadeh A, Mirzaee M, Farokhzadian J (2019) Professsional values of nurses and nursing students: a comparative study. BMC Med Educ 19:438. https://doi.org/10.1186/s12909-019-1878-2

Purc E, Laguna M (2019) Personal values and innovative behavior of employees. Front Psychol 10:865. https://doi.org/10.3389/fpsyg.2019.00865

Rath T, Conchie B (2008) Strengths based leadership. Gallup Press, New York

Rokeach M (1973) The nature of human values. Free Press, New York

Samson W (2009) The personal accountability revolution. The workplace development process. Workshop, 10. Podium presentation at the 2014 Wyoming Nurses Association Convention; 2014 September 18: Casper, Wyoming

Schober M (2017) Strategic planning for advanced nursing practice. Springer International, Basel

Shahriari M, Mohammadi E, Abbaszadeh A, Bahrami M (2013) Nursing ethical values and definitions: a literature review. Iran J Nurs Midwifery Res 18(1):1–8

Teoli D, An J (2020) SWOT analysis. In: StatPearls [Internet]. StatPearls Publishing, Treasure Island [Updated 2019 Jan 4]. https://www.ncbi.nlm.nih.gov/books/NBK537302/

The Human Memory. Memory Encoding (2019). https://human-memory.net/memory-encoding/. Accessed 24 Mar 2019

Toyoda S (2020) 5 whys: the ultimate root cause analysis tool. In: Kanbanize. https://kanbanize.com/lean-management/improvement/5-whys-analysis-tool. Accessed 9 Apr 2020

Tuulik K, Õunapuu T, Kuimet K, Titov E (2016) Rokeach's instrumental and terminal values as descriptors of modern organisation values. Int J Organ Leadersh 5:151–161. https://doi.org/10.33844/ijol.2016.60252

Vaismoradi M, Salsali M, Ahmadi F (2011) Perspective of Iranian male nursing students regarding the role of nursing education in developing a professional identity: a content analysis study. Jpn J Nurs Sci 8:174–183. https://doi.org/10.1111/j.1742-7924.2010.00172.x

von Kodolitsch Y, Bernhardt AM, Robinson N, Kölbel T, Reichenspurner H, Debus S, Detter C (2015) Analysis of strengths, weaknesses, opportunities, and threats as a tool for translating evidence into Individualized Medical Strategies (I-SWOT). Aorta 3(3):98–107. https://doi.org/10.12945/j.aorta.2015.14.064

Williams S (2002) Strategic planning and organizational values: links to alignment. Hum Resour Dev Int 5(2):217–233

Integrate Your Growing Professional Identity Within Your Role Transition

7

7.1 Introduction

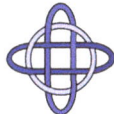

This final chapter aims to help a person understand the synergistic effects of developing a positive professional identity in order to follow a structured path to successful APN role transition. After graduation, APN students will be beginning the role as APN to provide advanced nursing including enhanced critical thinking, decision-making, diagnostic understanding, and provision of autonomous care. The result of your APN role transition is dependent upon many factors that are both personal (you have control) and environmental (you have no control over). This chapter provides you with insight on four competency domains which are impacted by both your professional identity and role transition. Lastly, this chapter (and book) concludes with a look forward after graduation and your workplace transition.

7.2 Definitions

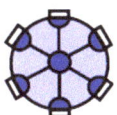

Competency A competency is specific knowledge or skill and the legal authority, ability, or admissibility to do the activity (https://www.merriam-webster.com/dictionary/competency accessed 22 April 2022).

© The Author(s), under exclusive license to Springer Nature Switzerland AG 2022   199
M. Kidner, *Successful Advanced Practice Nurse Role Transition*, Advanced
Practice in Nursing, https://doi.org/10.1007/978-3-030-53002-0_7

Domain A domain is a specified sphere of activity or knowledge (https://www. merriam-webster.com/dictionary/domain accessed 22 April 2022). As applied in this chapter, *domain* is specific to the specialized APN knowledge and activities associated with the APN role.

Forethought Forethought is the use of self-reflection to gain motivation, develop goals, create action plans, and visualize the outcomes of one's actions (Bandura 2018).

Intrapersonal Thoughts occurring within the individual mind or self (https:// www.merriam-webster.com/dictionary/intrapersonal accessed 22 April 2022). Intrapersonal is having to do with yourself and involves your self-concept and your ability to self-talk with the use of forethought (Bandura 2018).

Intraprofessional People in the same professional are intraprofessional (https:// medical-dictionary.thefreedictionary.com/intraprofessional+team accessed 22 April 2022). As applied in this book, intraprofessional is specific to the profession of nursing and includes all levels, or roles of nursing.

Interpersonal When two or more people come together the being, relating to, relationships and interactions between the persons are interpersonal (https://www. merriam-webster.com/dictionary/interpersonally accessed 22 April 2022).

Interprofessional Interprofessional is when two or more different professionals are working together (https://www.merriam-webster.com/dictionary/interprofessional accessed 22 April 2022). As applied to this book, interprofessional would include a wide range of healthcare professionals and stakeholders including nursing, physicians, formal leaders, respiratory therapist, physical therapists, dieticians, laboratory technicians, patients, community, and even outside professionals of engineers, public health, transportation specialists, or public communication professionals.

Paradigm A *paradigm* is a philosophical or theoretical framework of any kind (https://www.merriam-webster.com/dictionary/paradigm accessed 22 April 2022). Scientific paradigms frame research methodology, data collection, and interpretation research in addition to being highly influential in developing behaviors and attitudes of professional groups (Deliktas et al. 2019).

Megaparadigms Dominant paradigms of a profession are megaparadigms (Deliktas et al. 2019). Developing megaparadigms within a profession allows for clarification of the fundamental thesis statements of the profession and a better appreciation of the scope of scientific research pertaining to the profession. In nursing there are four megaparadigms: health, person, nursing, and environment (Deliktas et al. 2019).

Personal Paradigm   When applied as a personal paradigm, it is a group of ideas a person has about how something should be done, made, or thought about (Candy 1982). Your personal paradigm is your mental setting to help you to interpret, define, and engage in the world around you. Every person has different paradigms that influence how they interpret the world. The two primary types of personal paradigms are (1) paradigms that help you combined concept analyses of professional. These paradigms are influenced by your values; (2) paradigms that help you interpret the way things are shaped by realities. Evaluating your paradigms helps you become more open-minded to others' perceptions, and ultimately expand your own view of the world (Sinusoid 2021).

Professional Paradigm   A philosophical and theoretical framework of a scientific school or discipline within which theories, laws, and generalizations and the experiments performed in support of them are formulated (https://www.merriam-webster.com/dictionary/paradigm accessed 22 April 2022).

Paradigm shift   A *paradigm shift* occurs when there has been a change in development of knowledge, skills, process or when the usual way of thinking about or doing something is replaced by a new and different way (https://www.merriam-webster.com/dictionary/paradigm%20shift accessed 22 April 2022). As applied to this book, the paradigm shift is when the generalist nurse's nursing paradigm is changed through the graduate APN education allowing the nursing paradigm to encompass the APN role, attributes, characteristics, and professional identity.

7.3   Recognize There Is a Process

Role transition from expert nurse to novice APN can be a tumultuous event and create a challenging paradigm shift (Faraz 2016). Anxiety and insecurity can contribute to the stress of the APN student and can increase role confusion if there is poor role identity through the educational process (Thompson 2019; Trede 2012). APN students that are supported through the development of personal values and positive professional identity tend to have a higher sense of purpose, confidence, and engagement with the APN profession (Purc and Laguna 2019; Vaismoradi et al. 2011). In turn, as an engaged and empowered graduate student, there is an increased willingness to work on interprofessional teams and to be a role advocate (Vaismoradi et al. 2011). Recognition and understanding of an evidence-based process that APN graduate students can utilize to guide role transition is helpful. This book explores the concept analyses of APN role transition and professional identity to provide a greater understanding of the process a nurse can experience as they transition from a generalist nurse to APN. Below is a graphic model (Fig. 7.1) of the two combined concept analyses of professional identity and role transition.

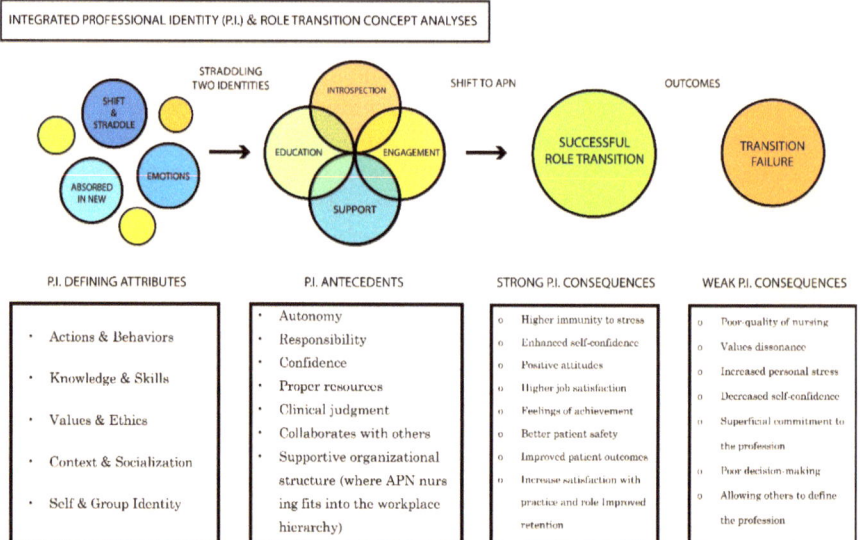

Fig. 7.1 Combined concept analyses: role transition + professional identity

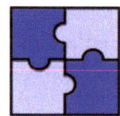

Review the combined concept analyses and write at least three aspects that relate to yourself.

_____
_____
_____
_____

7.4   Gain Self-Understanding Through Introspection

One aspect of being an effective APN as clinical expert, advocate, and mentor is to have a process to evaluate self to ensure you are providing the correct level of education or mentorship to others. You have spent time in forethought considering yourself, now it is time to consider your impact on your stakeholders. A process to evaluate your impact can be through the review of four APN *Competency Domains* (Kidner 2019). As an APN student you would primarily apply this section to yourself and to your patients as you implement your patient education and planned care.

As an APN you apply your integration of these competency domains through the viewpoint of clinical expertise and clinical leadership. These APN competency domains can be used to judge your impact on other people. This discussion concerning the APN competency domains in this chapter will be focused on clinical expertise. The sequel to this book focuses the APN competency domains on clinical leadership in formal and informal settings.

7.5   The Four APN Competency Domains

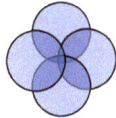

This book supports the use of four competency domains as skilled areas for APNs to develop and expand their social influence processes to be a positive influence for patients, peers, and community (Kidner 2019). The domains are four distinct, yet interrelated, processes that an APN utilizes daily.

The four distinct competency domains are:

1. **Relationships:** The ability to build trust relationships on interpersonal and intrapersonal levels.
2. Skills and Knowledge: The advanced nursing skills and knowledge needed to provide advance autonomous care.
3. **Thinking:** The ability and skills for critically and creative thinking leading to critical decision and creative innovations.
4. **Clinical Expertise:** Comprehensive clinical expertise as APN with positive role transition and strong professional identity. This competency includes individual and team settings (Kidner 2019).

The competencies within each domain are characterized by the skills and abilities, knowledge and experiences, attitudes and behaviors that are exhibited in professional APN practice. Each domain is impacted by the APN's knowledge, self-concept, professional identity, and the person's ability to overcome challenges for a successful role transition.

Conducting a self-review of each competency domain will help you understand yourself better in addition to providing you evidence of your impact upon your stakeholders. As an APN student you can review yourself in the context of novice to expert within each domain and monitor your progress as you journey through role transition. Each of the four domains will be discussed.

7.5.1   Relationships Domain

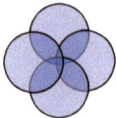

The relationship domain can also be called, "Emotional Intelligence." Your emotional intelligence is your collection of skills and abilities that allows you to assess and understand your own emotions, the emotions of others, and have the ability to appropriately respond with balanced stress management and adaptability (Mar Molero Jurado et al. 2019). This domain is about relationships, communication, and engagement with others. Relationships impact the health and well-being of people and different types of relationships (at home, at work, with friends, as a patient and others) influence every person in all other relationships. This domain is the most complicated domains because the main expectation is strong, trusting relationships and the goal is upholding values such as integrity, honesty, trustworthiness, accountability, and innovation.

There are two distinct levels of this relationship domain:

1. Personal level
2. Professional level

7.5.1.1 Personal Level of the Relationship Domain

There are two important types of relationships: Intrapersonal and Interpersonal (Chambers 2018; Oleś et al. 2020).

Intrapersonal   The activities of understanding yourself and the activities occurring within your mind which become the relationship with yourself is your intrapersonal relationship. Self-talk is ubiquitous in humans. Your self-monologue can create a positive or negative impact to self-image, thus self-efficacy and professional identity (Oleś et al. 2020).

Developing strong intrapersonal skills will allow you to improve in many skills that aid in your resiliency in times of change, challenges, and chaos. Table 7.1 provides possible activities a person can complete to improve intrapersonal skills.

Understanding yourself requires introspection and personal reflection to review one's self-concept in the context of the intrapersonal skills (above). Through a review of past and current events when considering the future allows a person to internalize and build personal values (Scott 2009; Kolorotius and Wessler 2007; Mar Molero Jurado et al. 2019). APNs with strong intrapersonal skills have better coping strategies and less burnout as these skills influence your ability to succeed with the daily high demands and stress (Mar Molero Jurado et al. 2019).

Your intrapersonal skills and awareness are your guides in considering ethical situations plus the building and evolution of your professional identity and self-concept. New knowledge and experiences are constantly compared to your paradigm and adjustments are made (Ackerman 2020). Establishing a daily habit of

Table 7.1 Intrapersonal skills and steps

Intrapersonal skill	The skills' outcome	Steps I can take
Self-concept	The ability to know yourself	• Determine your strengths through a SWOT (refer to Chap. 6) • Recognize and celebrate your increases in skills, knowledge, decision-making as your education increases • Review feedback and support provided to become better • Determine your personal values and use them daily (refer to Chap. 6) • See yourself in a positive and healthy light • Take responsibility for your choices and actions • Acknowledge your uniqueness
Assertiveness/ initiative	The ability to start change or take the lead	• Request and provide feedback • Request a mentor and be a dedicated mentee • Volunteer to lead a project • Be active in team meetings—offer evidence-based suggestions • Be self-directed and actively consider new and creative processes • Build and use a personal strategic plan (refer to Chap. 6)
Learning/ unlearning	The ability to change	• Determine a new skill or knowledge you want to achieve and implement a process to achieve it. • Recognize you may need to unlearn and old process/ knowledge and accept a new process • Practice to gain a consistent habit of the new skill or knowledge
Adaptability	The ability to be resilient	• Increase your job autonomy • Get and use constructive feedback • Listen to others—be open-minded • Try something new (take a risk of volunteering to a new role, or new task) • Accept multiple perspectives • Have good evidence-based references/knowledge to support the change • Be an early adaptor to well-planned and evidence-based change • Be consistent in action and voice
Emotional maturity	The ability to think before responding	• Reframe your thoughts of a problem from pessimistic to optimistic • Identify your emotional triggers and develop a plan to control your maladaptive emotions • Consider and anticipate the emotions of others • Recognize and celebrate your positive emotions • Show respect and attention to the needs of others • Develop a habit of self-talk to develop a healthy intrapersonal communication

(continued)

Table 7.1 (continued)

Intrapersonal skill	The skills' outcome	Steps I can take
Self-efficacy	The ability for autonomous success	• Believe in your capabilities, knowledge, and skills • Ask for feedback to guide and build confidence • Watch others to gain vicarious experiences • Work hard to gain mastery of skills, knowledge, and decision-making • Maintain your integrity to develop trust relationships
Stress management	The ability to look after oneself	• Take physical care of yourself through healthy lifestyle management • Self-review for unhealthy or inappropriate habits and replace them with healthy behaviors • Develop a creative hobby • Have a support friend or mentor with whom you can share your emotions, fears, worries, and joys • Review your passions and set time to grow your passion • Develop good work/school and life (family and self) time
Professional identity	The ability to understand, engage, and embody the attributes of the profession into daily activities	• Know the APN role, the scope of practice, sociopolitical processes, and regulation in your country • Know and embody the attributes of the APN role and practice • Embrace forethought, feedback, and scholarly discussion on ethics, decision-making, and judgment-based practice • Know your values and maintain integrity to your values • Gain the required APN graduate educational and clinical experiences for advanced practice nursing

Anderson et al. (2020), Bandura (2018), Branch and George (2017), Dickert and Kass (2009), Ewertsson et al. (2017), Ibrahim et al. (2017), Johnson et al. (2012), Kidner (2019), Oleś et al. (2020), Parschau et al. (2013), Trede (2012)

3–5 min daily to review your day and decisions made would be advantageous to a smooth role transition and understanding of professional identity growth.

Intrapersonal Habit Formation

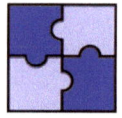

1. Choose a witnessed event or decision you made in the past:

_____

_____

2. Self-introspection: Ask yourself these questions:

_____

_____

Did this event/decision go as I thought it
should have gone? Why?

Did this event/decision show me
something of myself I did not
anticipate? What?

Was I assertive during this event/
decision? What should I do the same if
this occurs again? What do I do
different?
What did I learn from this event/
decision?

Do I need to adapt my thinking,
planning, or actions for a similar event?

What emotions did I feel during and
after this event/decision? Do I need to
change my response for a similar event?

If this event/decision occurs again, how
would I respond to it on my own?

Was this event/decision stressful? What
should I do about the stress?

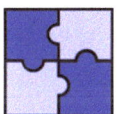

Intrapersonal Activity   Review the intrapersonal components and rate yourself
where you feel you are today on each component.

Intrapersonal components	Self-rate novice to expert (place X on continuum)				
	Novice	Adv beginner	Competent	Proficient	Expert
Self-awareness	I_____I				
Adaptability	I_____I				
Stress management	I_____I				
Emotional maturity	I_____I				
Taking the initiative	I_____I				
Learning and unlearning	I_____I				
Self-efficacy	I_____I				

Consider your current self-review, write at least two positive steps you can achieve to develop a healthy intrapersonal relationship.

Notes: _____

_____

_____

_____

_____

Interpersonal being, relating to, or involving relations between persons (https://www.merriam-webster.com/dictionary/interpersonal?src=search-dict-hed). It is the relationships we have with others.

Developing strong skills for interpersonal relationships requires time, work, and practice. Just recognizing the different aspects of communications and understanding how one currently uses these skills will provide direction for improvement. There are many aspects to excellent communications.

Activity In this personal activity, determine your current ability concerning some aspects of interpersonal relationships.

Rate yourself from 0 = no ability to 2 = Average ability to 4 = excellent ability

• Caring	0	1	2	3	4
• Communicating (written and verbal) clearly	0	1	2	3	4
• Active listening	0	1	2	3	4
• Managing conflict	0	1	2	3	4
• Dialogue	0	1	2	3	4
• Facilitating	0	1	2	3	4
• Partnering	0	1	2	3	4
• Collaborating	0	1	2	3	4
• Directing, guiding, and delegating	0	1	2	3	4
• Providing constructive feedback	0	1	2	3	4
• Receptive to negative feedback	0	1	2	3	4
• Understanding diversity	0	1	2	3	4
• Teamwork	0	1	2	3	4
• Positive attitude	0	1	2	3	4

Consider your current self-review, write at least two positive steps you can achieve to develop a healthy interpersonal relationships.

Notes: _____

_____

_____

_____

_____

This self-review is to increase your awareness of the relationship competency domain. As an APN student you can focus on yourself and how you build relationships with friends, staff, peers, and patients. This activity can provide you with insight to your strengths and weaknesses concerning your ability and impact of developing trust relationship with everyone you will impact.

7.5.1.2 The Professional Relationship Aspect of the Relationship Domain

The second aspect of this domain concerns the intraprofessional and interprofessional relationships that are required for effective high-quality healthcare.

Intraprofessional Relationships

Intraprofessional relationships are those relationships within all levels of nursing. Building strong relationships with all levels of nursing helps to shape the public and stakeholder view of the nursing role, education, and outcomes. As APN you can improve your intraprofessional relationships by the following activities:

- Verbally support, encourage, and thank nurses publicly
- Offer to provide topic education that could help bedside nurses understand and improve their care
- Offer to mentor other nurses
- Provide constructive feedback

Interprofessional Relationships

Interprofessional relationships are those connection made working in multidisciplinary groups and teams. Healthy interprofessional relationships take time to build trust that allows each person to be free to share ideas and feedback. As APN you can improve your interprofessional relationships by the following activities:

- Role clarity for every profession in group/team
- Encourage active participation of each person by upholding dignity and respect for ideas and feedback
- Use evidence-based practices and research to support your actions and contributions to the group
- Provide constructive feedback

Seek to understand the point of view of every team member

7.5.2 Knowledge and Skills Domain

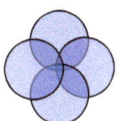

This domain is perhaps the most exciting aspect of becoming an APN. There are two distinct aspects of this domain: knowledge and skills. As an APN, your skills and specialized clinical knowledge will be built upon your nursing foundations, enhanced by your graduate education, and strengthened through your clinical experiences. Gaining and understanding the technical knowledge is required for APNs to provide safe, effective, and excellent care (Von Collin-Appling and Giuliano 2017).

As an APN student, you can use this competency domain to self-assess and to assess your patient's knowledge and/or skills required to safely provide self-care. To help your patient achieve success you should be assessing your patient's family, or support people's knowledge and skills to implement the healthcare, medication plans, and lifestyle management you are prescribing. These assessments will include the knowledge and skills needed for your patient and their support people to make an improvement in their health and wellness. As a practicing APN you will also be using the knowledge and skills competency domain to evaluate, coach, and provide the accurate level of education to staff and peers.

7.5.2.1 Knowledge

In your graduate education, you are gaining knowledge specific to human anatomy, psychology, physiology, and pathology that is manifested in diagnostic and physical data. Your decisions of pharmaceuticals and prescribed treatment care plans are based upon your knowledge. This information is obtained through your formal education and clinical experiences and will continue daily through your career.

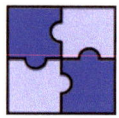

In the area you want to be employed as an APN, what area of specific knowledge do you want to grow or maintain as a clinical expert in your future clinical practice?

_____
_____
_____
_____

7.5.2.2 Skills

As an APN, you will learn specialized skills required for your expanded nursing role. Some of these skills may include setting splints and casts, suturing, and advance trauma skills (such as intubation, chest tubes, ultrasound, 12-lead EKGs, and central line placement). Each new skill takes time and mentorship to become an expert.

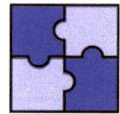

Activity When looking forward to your APN clinical practice, you will recognize that there are several additional skills APNs can provide. This exercise is to help you identify skills you have and may need in the future.

What advanced skills can you do now? _____
_____
_____

What advanced skills do you want to learn? _____
_____
_____

7.5.3   Creative and Critical Thinking Domain

7.5.3.1 Thinking Is a Learned Skill!

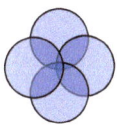

This competency domain is focused on decision-making abilities. "Thinking" is a process of reasoning by using your knowledge and past experiences to make decisions. The two types of thinking in this domain are: critical and creative thinking. Critical thinking often involves breaking a complex problem into small solvable problems. Creative thinking is the ability to have a new idea, or a new way to try to solve a problem. Creativity focuses on the possibility that there is more than one way to solve a problem. To be a successful APN, you will need to practice both thinking processes of critical and creative thinking.

7.5.3.2 Critical Thinking

APNs are impacting healthcare in communities, clinics, and hospitals. In addition, APNs are making direct healthcare decisions, implementing new policies, leading change, conducting research, and mentoring others. These activities are dependent upon a person's ability to think critically. There are four steps of critical thinking:

Step 1. Knowledge acquisition and application of knowledge
Step 2. The analysis of information—the balance between perception and reality
Step 3. The process of informed decision-making
Step 4. Reflection—the review of process, or debriefing after a process, event, or
decision (Von Collin-Appling and Giuliano 2017)

Critical thinking is a process about how you think, assess your knowledge and abilities, and regulate your decisions. Much of your professional identity is developed through a critical thinking process by reviewing what you have learned in didactic education and compare those truths to your experience to determine the ethics and evidence-based practice level of the situation (Ewertsson et al. 2017).

A risk management foundation on diagnostics reported in 75% of cases of errors of diagnosing, poor critical thinking skills contributed to the error (Hayes et al. 2017). Therefore, it is important to review your critical decision-making skills and to actively pursue strategies to improve.

Activity Below is a list of skills that aid critical thinking. Place a mark where you feel your current level of ability is at for each skill. As you gain education, experience, and confidence, your novice to expert level should increase. This self-review is only a guide for you to recognize skills that you can use to increase your critical thinking.

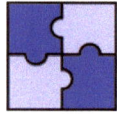

Critical Thinking Skills

	Novice	Expert
• Planning	I_____I	
• Evaluating and analyzing	I_____I	
• Problem-solving	I_____I	
• Decision-making	I_____I	
• Priority-setting	I_____I	
• Allocating resources: time-people-money-equipment	I_____I	
• A reflecting practice	I_____I	
• Learning	I_____I	
• Change management	I_____I	
• Probability analysis	I_____I	
• Ethical decision-making	I_____I	

Hayes et al. (2017), Koloroutis and Wessler (2007)

7.5.3.3 Creative Thinking

Being creative in the health field is important when seeking new ways to complete tasks, use resources, provide care, implement training programs, or change behavior. Creativity is the generation of something both different and useful (Beaty et al. 2016). Brainstorming, developing graphic models, or using brain maps are all aspects of creative thinking. Creative thinking involves dynamic interactions of large-scale brain systems and supports complex cognitive processes. Goal-directed and self-generated thought is a key component of creative thinking (Beaty et al. 2016).

Creative Thinking Skills There are a variety of skills that can aid creativity. Table 7.2 provides eleven different creative thinking skills to consider and be inspired to become more creativity in your professional life.

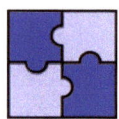

Table 7.2 Creative thinking skills

Creative thinking skill	Explanation/implementing suggestions
Generating ideas	**A process to generate ideas can include:** • Group meetings to discuss the concern/issue. • Completing a SWOT analysis on the topic. • Ask "What would you do?" to people outside your department. • Conduct a group process to discuss an issue through a brain map or graphic model.
Synthesizing	**Taking different parts of other solutions and create a new solution:** • Seek similar concerns/problems and review all solutions, then work in group for possibilities • Look to other industry or department for solutions
Stretching boundaries	**Review the current boundaries of the topic, then remove the boundaries and ask what could be done if the boundary/barrier was removed**. • Do in groups, as questionnaire, or group SWOT. • Have small groups answer a problem through the use of a graphic model, or brain map. • Always provide support that stretching boundaries is good to assess innovation.
New patterns and possibilities	**Review current patterns of the process, culture, and outcomes** • Determine the current process, culture, or outcome, then identify the desired process, culture, or outcome. • Seek information from a wide source of people. • Build the new way.
Suspended judgment	• Allow every idea to be discussed and considered important. • Seek input from every stakeholder. • Actively listen and support every idea to see which idea become the best fit for the solution. • Do not let another person's idea to be dismiss or berated in group discussions. • Seek consensus and not majority.
Novelty	• Consider teaching in a new way, implementing a new idea/product in a different way from tradition. • Look to other industries for solutions or ideas. • Be open-minded • Seek all assumptions and discuss every assumption to then consider a new idea.
Creating	Allowing innovation thinking. • Have the involved team member use graphic models to express ideas and thoughts on the topic. • Have a creative contest to solve the current concern. • Provide a short creative activity before the formal meeting (write a poem, draw, use blocks to build, complete a puzzle).
Divergent thinking	• Allowing all possibilities to be looked at • Use large pieces of paper and write all ideas down. • Conduct group activities where ideas build. • Include all ideas (suspend judgment)

(continued)

Table 7.2 (continued)

Creative thinking skill	Explanation/implementing suggestions
Learning	**Gaining knowledge and skill**
	• Provide the inspiration, infrastructure (supplies and resources).
	• Provide the correct training level from novice to expert for the team.
	• Have the team teach each other.
	• Include engaging activities in the training.
	• Have the team determine training topics.
Strategic thinking	**Looking to future and how new ideas would look**
	• Consider the impact of innovative ideas to all stakeholders.
	• Review the values and build behavior changes to support the values.
	• Work in groups/teams to project the future and present.
Leading change	**Providing support, coaching, and mentoring to implement change**
	• Involve and support those who will be active in the change process.
	• Present change as the desired outcome of the team
	• Develop at least two different platforms of presentation (such as written, graphic model, oral presentation).
	• Teach mentorship skills.
	• Decrease the perceived negative impact of the change to stakeholders (such as nurses perceive a change will add more duties and time to their already stressed days).
	• Seek consensus and understanding the thoughts of those who oppose the change.

Bacal (n.d.) accessed 4 Feb 2020, Beaty et al. (2016), Branch and George (2017), Dickert and Kass (2009), Katz (2018), Koloroutis and Wessler (2007), Millick (2012), Roberto (2011)

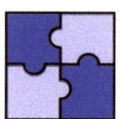

Activity Describe a decision you made or activity you completed that you felt was creative. Explain what made it creative. If you can work in a small group, share in small groups and discuss creativity and its impact on decisions, activities, or integrating new processes in the workplace.

_____
_____
_____
_____
_____
_____
_____
_____

Creative Activity Choose a current topic from your APN education and build a graphic model to explain the topic and then share your graphic with another person to ascertain the effectiveness of your graphic.

Ethical Decisions

Ethical decisions will require both sets of thinking skills: creative and critical. APNs will need to know the nurse's codes of ethics within their country, local policies, organizational policies, and the evidence-based standards of care to make good decision concerning ethical dilemmas (Barlow et al. 2018). There is an overlap of the domains with relationships, knowledge/skill, and decision-making which are required to assess and determine an action in ethical dilemmas.

7.5.4 Clinical Expertise Domain

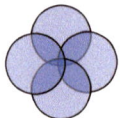

The clinical expertise domain is centered upon the primary components of highly successful APNs: clinical expertise, informal leadership abilities, mentor abilities, and highly functional in interprofessional teamwork. As an APN student you can use this clinical expertise domain for self-reflection on your current capacity of translating your didactic knowledge combined with your communication abilities to guide, mentor, and coach others. As an APN, you can use this domain to understand and develop your clinical impact of informal and formal leadership through your clinical expertise (Kidner 2019).

Developing clinical expertise is the summation process of your role transition, having a positive self-concept, an excellent understanding of the APN role and scope of practice, and strong professional identity. There are several key components of APN clinical practice where this domain is central to achievement including:

- Being autonomous and accountable at an advanced nursing level
- Provides safe and competent patient care through a designated APN role or level of nursing
- Applies the theoretical and clinical skills of advanced practice
- Works as a consultant to nurses and other healthcare professionals in managing complex patient care problems
- Influences advanced practice nursing through leadership, education, research, and policy
- Provides evidence-based care and supports nurses and other healthcare professionals to provide evidence-based care
- Recognizes limitations and maintains clinical competencies through continued professional development
- Adheres to the ethical standards of nursing
- Identifies and initiate required diagnostic test and procedures
- Gathers and interprets assessment data to formulate plan of care
- Completes excellent clinical documentation written and verbal reports
- Performs specialty-specific procedures
- Assesses patient or family response to therapy and modifies plan of care on the basis of response
- Communicates plan of care and response to patient and family
- Provides appropriate education to patient and family

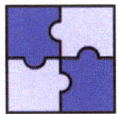

Activity Clinical expertise encompasses far more than advanced knowledge and skills. To be a clinical expert, you need the skills to share your knowledge through word and action. Below are some personal actions/knowledge that are beneficial to prove your clinical expertise as APN. What level from Novice to Expert are you in each area? Place a mark on each continuum where you think you are now.

	Novice	Competent	Expert
• Being a role model	I_____I		
• Being creative	I_____I		
• Be caring	I_____I		
• Be affirming	I_____I		
• Be encouraging	I_____I		
• Being present	I_____I		
• Using skills to show knowledge	I_____I		
• Giving honest feedback	I_____I		
• Developing trust	I_____I		
• Using knowledge for decisions	I_____I		
• Know your strengths, work styles, and values	I_____I		
• Having a positive self-concept	I_____I		
• Knowledge of APN Scope of Practice	I_____I		

Review the above skills/knowledge and write about at least two that you can develop that will help show others your clinical expertise in providing autonomous clinical practice.

_____
_____
_____
_____
_____
_____
_____

7.5.4.1 Professional Identity and Professionalism

APN professional identity is related to the common knowledge, skills, behaviors, and values that are shared by APNs worldwide and obtained through a socialization process (Owens 2019). As knowledge and skills advance through research and technology so will the professional identity change to reflect new wisdom. Each APN develops a professional identity of who they are as APN based upon the combination of their personal identity, the development of new knowledge, their experiences of role transition and then APN practice (Owens 2019). Both self-concept and professional identity are moldable as they develop and change over time due to experiences and change in knowledge of both the profession and of self (Trede 2012).

Role transition is facilitated when there is a formal process to allow students to gain the knowledge, skills, and ethics as needed for the APN role (Owens 2019). Students who can articulate the rationale for their actions and decisions develop a strong ethical balance and develop a stronger professional identity (Trede et al. 2011). The formal process involves a planned post-clinical/traumatic event review and discussion with peers, mentors, clinical preceptors, or professors.

Professional identity development includes the past, present, and future of one's experiences, knowledge, skills, and ability to make decisions that are based on the past habits with conscious thought towards the future. As a person understands oneself, they develop higher levels of self-assurance and self-confidence (Branch and George 2017; Owens 2019; Trede 2012). One's self-concept is then tied to a profession (Goliroshan et al. 2021). The APN role is interwoven with the responsibility, accountability, and authority one has in making judgments and decisions based upon APN knowledge and scope of practice. The process and acts of being, thinking, and acting as a professional within the realm of the APN role are your underpinnings of APN professionalism and a sense of professional identity within the APN community.

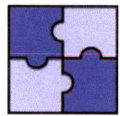

A deep sense of professional attachment can be developed through the membership in nursing organizations.

Are there nursing organizations/associations in your country (local, national, or international)?

_____

Which APN professional organizations/associations can or do you belong to (local, national, or international):

_____

Which health or public organizations do you want to belong (local, national, or international) to promote nursing, the APN role, and health/wellness? _____

_____

Your personal professional identity will change over the years with your life's experiences and changes in knowledge/technology. Yet, there are some similarities within the timeline of professional identity (Barone et al. 2019). Table 7.3 splits the role transition into student, new graduate to 24 months, and later in APN practice and provides typical activities and professional identity milestones to provide an overall understanding of the potential growth of your professional identity.

Table 7.3 Timeline and professional identity activities

Professional timeline	Professional identity activities. The APN…
As a student	• Follows the rules and perceived social norms of the role.
	• Is impacted by professors, preceptors, and clinical practice sites.
	• Appreciates other's viewpoint, yet the focus is on self-views.
As a new graduate to 12–24 months	• Gains insight on APN practice through multiple perspectives.
	• Considers other's viewpoint strongly to compare with self-view and may change their personal viewpoint.
	• Has a sense of belonging to the APN role, but may not feel truly "professional."
	• May still have trouble with competing expectations, role ambiguity, and workload.
Later in APN Practice	• Seeks and understands differing values and perspectives.
	• Is engaged and accountable to the expectations of the role locally, nationally and maybe even globally.
	• Internalizes personal and professional values that motivate and inspire healthy habits in others.
	• Reconciles challenges between personal and professional expectations more effectively.
	• Able to expand time and expertise on policy and mentoring the APN role locally, nationally and maybe even globally.

Barone et al. (2019)

7.5.4.2 Self-Assessment on Your Professional Identity Development Level

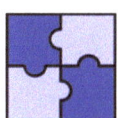

	Need help		OK		Doing great
I feel confident I understand the APN role	1	2	3	4	5
I feel connected to the APN role	1	2	3	4	5
I feel that I can be an APN advocate	1	2	3	4	5
I can explain the APN role/activities to others	1	2	3	4	5
I understand the APN role in my country	1	2	3	4	5
I have a person I can talk ethics to when needed	1	2	3	4	5

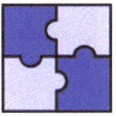

Write a 1–3 action plans (Chap. 6) for any above activity that you rated as a 1 or 2 level.

_____

_____

Professional status is a privilege, and in some countries, nursing may not be considered a "profession." Yet, every nurse can work on professionalism every day. As mentioned before, professionalism must be taught, supported, and mentored to reach its full potential of impact on APN students, faculty, patients, and all stakeholders. If the educational process includes the incorporation of values and characteristics of professionalism in all aspects of the educational experience, then what are the characteristics of the APN profession? Below is a list compiled from the review of this book that have been discussed and considered attributes of the APN profession. Circle the attributes that you embody.

Characteristics of the APN profession

- Altruism
- Autonomy
- Caring and compassion
- Commitment
- Competence
- Confidentiality
- Evidence-based knowledge/skill
- Insight
- Integrity and honesty
- Innovation and creativity
- Listening
- Moral and ethical conduct
- Mutually agreed plans
- Openness
- Presence
- Respect and honor the patient
- Responsibility to the profession
- Responsibility to society
- Teamwork

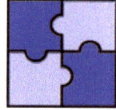

Activity In team of 3–5 people, choose (or make up) a recent dilemma from someone's clinical experience. Discuss each of the above APN attributes and discuss how they relate to the understanding, impact, or solving the dilemma. This activity can be completed as individuals.

_____
_____
_____
_____
_____
_____
_____
_____
_____

7.5.4.3 Other Supports

Psychologist Albert Bandura's life's work has been in human behavior and social cognitive theory. He developed the agentic theory in which the interplay of personal, behavioral, and environmental determinants become the product of human activity. People can affect their lives individually, by a proxy (society), or within a group. A group working towards a common cause that can share knowledge, skills, resources, and support can collectively help the group achieve the common purpose (Bandura 2018). Within your setting of your graduate program, developing friendships with fellow students to become a group with a common purpose (graduation and successful APN role transition) can become a strong support system to share and discuss experiences, and dreams of the future. Many of these supportive relationships will become lifelong friendships.

List your fellow students whom you want to be their support person to help them through their graduate education:

_____

Write at least one SMART action plan (see Chap. 6) for you to support a fellow student.

_____
_____
_____
_____

You will find when you reach out to provide support to another peer, you also gain an insight on your self-concept and self-efficacy as you grow in the share trust relationship of peer friendship through the sharing of common fears, anxiety, stress, knowledge, and even joys.

7.6   A Second Role Transition: Going from APN Student to APN in the Workplace

So far, this book has been focused on your current activities of graduate education and role transition. However, once you graduate you will have to enter the workplace as an APN. After-graduation role transition can be at its highest level of uncertainty, fear, curiosity, and challenges at the time of clinical practice entry. Yet, at this point you have also been developing your confidence and self-concept through formation of your professional identity. Plus, you have developed a personalized role transition strategic plan in which you developed your values, vision, mission, goals, and action plans for a successful transition. It is wise to understand your next role transition process that occurs after graduation as an APN with the understanding that the consequences of significant transitions have an effect on your self-concept and professional identity.

There is research concerning the process of role transition after graduation for many professions. These studies identify a distinct time from graduation to job obtainment through the first year of work to be emotional, stressful, and challenging including the possibility of feeling like an imposter (Ares 2018; Brown and Olshansky 1997; Graf et al. 2020; Gottlieb et al. 2020; Heitz et al. 2004; Owens 2019; Poronsky 2013). This author has chosen two ways to prospectively look at your future as an APN graduate: (1) based on working through a process of self-awareness (Limbo to Legitimacy) and (2) the use of an estimated time frame of transition.

7.6.1   A Process of Self-Awareness: *Limbo to Legitimacy* Theory

This theory was initially presented in 1997 by Marie-Annette Brown and Ellen F. Olshansky. Although this theory was developed decades ago, it has stood the test of time and remains relevant today. Graduation from your APN graduate student role is the time you will take on your new professional role. This is a defining moment in your life and role transition. Your professional identity, your self-concept and your self-efficacy are your support systems to help you travel your next 1–2 years as APN. According to this theory, there are four stages that occur post-graduation as an APN transitions from student to APN clinical provider (see Fig. 7.2):

- **Stage I** is called *"Laying the foundation."* This stage occurs from graduation to the day the APN starts their APN job. This is the timeframe in which a new APN first recuperates from having completed a graduate advanced nursing education and then works on the process of obtaining an APN job. This timeframe tends to remain unsettling with high levels of worry of both finding a job and having the ability to function as a competent APN. Some students will push this stage to before the actual graduation as they seek a job during the final months of their graduate program. The key process to achieve is recuperation and rejuvenation from the rigors of graduate APN education. Although this process has worry as a primary emotion, the recuperation allows the new APN to gain the energy and engagement for the next stage (Brown and Olshansky 1997).

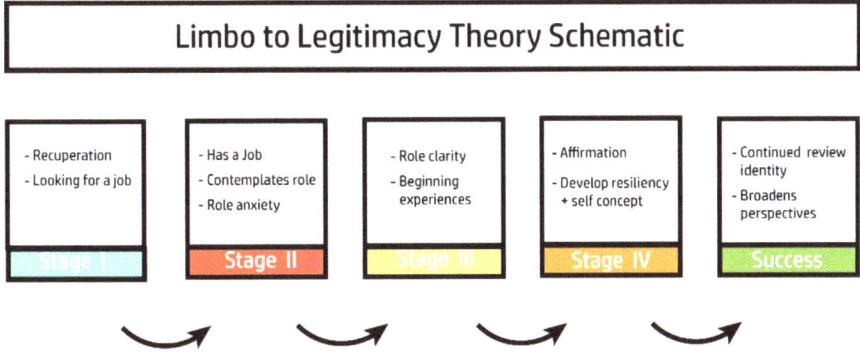

Fig. 7.2   Schematic of the *Limbo to Legitimacy* theory (Brown and Olshansky 1997)

- **Stage II** is called "*Launching*." This stage is when the new APN has started their first job as APN. Most often there is high anxiety as the new graduate confronts the reality and responsibility of the new APN role which is markedly different from their previous nursing job. The process of launching is often difficult as the new APN is required to overcome their lack of experience with subsequent recognition that they can provide high-quality advanced nursing care. It is within this stage that the imposter phenomenon can occur (Brown and Olshansky 1997).

Imposter Phenomenon (IP)

A common challenge faced after graduation is the *Imposter Phenomenon* (or syndrome) (Ares 2018; Brown and Olshansky 1997; Gottlieb et al. 2020; Mullangi and Jagsi 2019). The imposter phenomenon (IP) occurs when a person has a sense of being an imposter working as a professional. As a psychological phenomenon, IP refers to a pattern of behavior where the person (even those with past success and graduation from a university) doubts their abilities and has a persistent fear of being exposed as a fraud (Mullangi and Jagsi 2019).

The most common time of development of IP is when starting a new profession or role. The development of IP occurs through a change in perception of one's self-efficacy and self-concept whereby the person becomes unable to recognize any workplace successes due to their personal activities or involvement (Gottlieb et al. 2020). The impact of IP can be devastating due to its high emotional impact. Medical residents reported 20–60% of all medical residents experiencing some aspects of IP (Gottlieb et al. 2020). Prevalence of IP on CNS role transition was 74% in a study involving 113 participants (Ares 2018). Research on role transitions support a time of confusion and fear when new APNs are transitioning into the reality of practice and are overwhelmed by the number of patients, complexity of care, and the need for clinical diagnosis. Thus, the risk of IP is high for new APNs.

IP links self-worth to achievement in a negative way where the person cannot recognize their personal achievements with the onset of IP occurring during significant times of professional change. Those at highest risk for IP are noted to be:

- Females
- High achievers
- Those who desire perfection
- Those with low self-concept
- Those experiencing inequities (Gottlieb et al. 2020; Mullangi and Jagsi 2019)

- **Stage III** is called "*Meeting the challenge*." This stage is where the new APN continues the process of role clarity and understanding their enhanced responsibility, accountability, and authority within their workplace. It is a time of increasing competence and confidence and is supported through peer mentorship and organizational support or even a formal process with the hallmark the development of a clear picture of themselves. The emotions of job stress and role transition decrease as confidence increases (Brown and Olshansky 1997).
- **Stage IV** is called "*Broadening the perspective*." This stage occurs when the new APN affirms oneself within the profession and within the organization as an effective APN. The process to achieve is the expansion of clinical attention from tasks and specific patients to recognition of systems and the seeking of new challenges to impact the workplace. There is continued development of the APN role and impact within teams, the workplace, and professional organizations. Success is built upon self-resiliency, stress management, time management, and organizational support structures (Brown and Olshansky 1997).

7.6.2   The Use of an Estimated Time Frame of Transition

Your APN role transition after completion of your graduate program into the workplace is a nonlinear process comprised of your experiences, role preparation and understanding, skill/knowledge changes, and role relationship changes (Duchscher 2008). The experiences and their meanings are compared to your expectations and anticipations. Although complex, there is predictability in this aspect of role transition. Duchscher (2008) developed the stages of transition theory for nurses which has three main stages that have a typical time to achievement. Although initially written for generalist nursing, this transition theory can be applied to APN transition from generalist nurse to an APN in the clinical setting. The three stages are *doing, being,* and *knowing* (see Fig. 7.3). Within each stage there are possible activities that you can experience to gain confidence in self, your knowledge, skills, and decision-making. Time is impacted by the support, orientation, and mentorship you may have in your workplace the first 12–18 months of your APN clinical practice. Transition

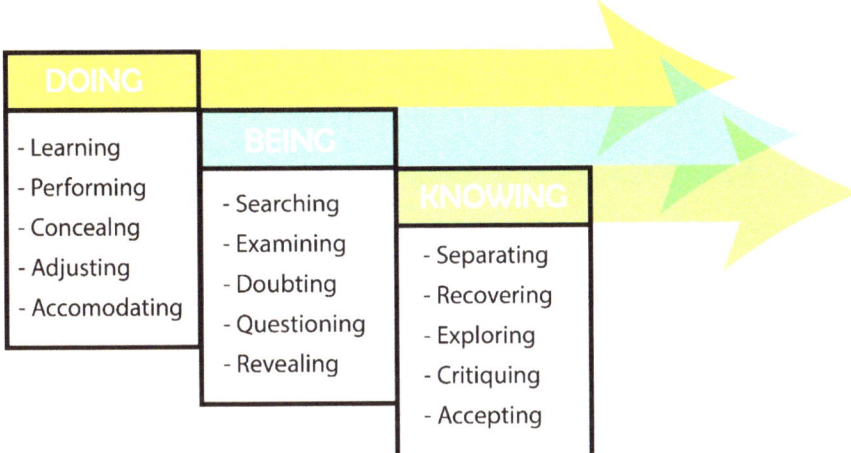

Fig. 7.3 A transition schematic based on the *Stages of Transition* Theory (Duchscher 2008)

support in formal orientation or mentorship has a positive outcome in role transition with greater confidence and competence (Dumphy et al. 2019; Hussein et al. 2017; Russell and Juliff 2021).

Stage I Doing: Months 0 to 3–4
- This stage is exemplified by the activities required to transition from the predictability of academic life to the chaos of change, new expectations, responsibilities, and level of accountability on the new role. This stage is filled with conflicting expectations between self and workplace. Most new APNs are surprised about the heavy patient workloads, and many suffered lateral and vertical abuse during this time (Duchscher 2008). Imposter phenomenon can occur during this time. Common emotions are self-doubt, wavering confidence, anxiety, and confusion. Yet, there is progress towards clinical competence (Russell and Juliff 2021).

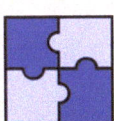

Steps to Overcome the Imposter Phenomenon
1. If you are a high-achiever, female, or have had previous feelings of IP, then recognize that IP is a distinct possibility and be ready with a plan.

2. If you find your intrapersonal communications to be negative, then take time to initiate your plan:

   (a) Have an identified trusted colleague you can share your thought and emotions about your current status in providing autonomous APN care.

   (b) Review this book and your APN education and write ten positive points concerning your success in school.

   - _____
   - _____
   - _____
   - _____
   - _____
   - _____
   - _____
   - _____
   - _____
   - _____

   (c) Review your recent activities in your APN and identify your contributions to correct diagnosis, interpretation for labs/testing, good plans for lifestyle management, and effective medication plans.

   (d) If you continue to suffer from IP, please seek support and help.

Stage II Being: Months 4 to 7–9

- This stage is exemplified by a rapid change in critical thinking, time management, and fulfilling the expected role. There is a waning in the negative emotions and there are the beginnings of trust relationships forming (Duchscher 2008). Yet, a lack of confidence, feeling of being placed to care for patients beyond the APN's clinical competence, and advanced responsibilities dominate the first months of the stage. However, reaching months 7–9, there is often a shift to the recognition that competent care can be provided, complex decisions can be made, and the knowledge and skills gained from graduate education were appropriate. The transition from the *Being stage* into the *Knowing stage* is marked by a rejuvenated professional identity and positive self-concept with enhanced self-efficacy through professional socialization and increased applied competence (Russell and Juliff 2021).

Stage III Knowing: Months 9–18

- This *Knowing stage* marks the successful role transition when the APN is fully accepted into the workplace. Trust relationships, self-confidence, and accountability are enhanced. There is increased autonomous care, and the APN can provide assistance and support to other team members. In this stage there is a renewed effort to understand and develop one's professional identity (Duchsher

2008). Figure 7.3 provides a graphic representation of the linear process of doing which leads into being which subsequently develops into knowing and successful role transition with confidence in the workplace and self.

7.6.3   Be Proactive

If you focus on the potential negatives, challenges, and stress of APN role transition, you can become overwhelmed. However, your capacity of learning and work performance is deeply embedded in your ability to be introspective of yourself, recognize your self-efficacy, self-concept, and define your personal competences (Grosemans et al. 2020). There are several activities you can do to be proactive to decrease role transition stresses, imposter phenomenon, and overcome challenges.

- Acknowledge change is hard and you are going through significant changes.
- Develop a personal transition strategic plan.
- Recognize your strengths and opportunities from your SWOT.
- Use reflective journaling and discuss the challenges you are facing and all of the knowledge and skills that you do well.
- Celebrate every clinic success (when you correctly understand and interpret a test, make a diagnosis, see improvement from your medication/treatment plan).
- Stay true to your values.
- Seek a categorical mentor for your clinical practice and role transition.
- Review your self-concept, self-efficacy, and professional identity weekly.
- Seek and fully participate in a workplace orientation.
- Develop your outside (non-workplace people) supports with family and friends and share with them the role transition process. Ask for their support and time to listen to you.
- Recognize that your patient assessments and diagnosis process will be slower for your first 6–12 months. This is normal.
- If you have feelings of being an imposter, share your feelings and thoughts with your mentor or trusted friend.
- Be aware of imposter phenomenon. If you find yourself unable to see your success and believe your diagnosis is "lucky," then reexamine your self-efficacy and all past successes. Seek support.
- Be prepared to succinctly explain your APN and scope of practice, and your clinical responsibilities.
- Be prepared for jealousy.
- Be aware of passive aggressive actions and have a plan on your response.
- Be committed to interprofessional collaboration and networking. Build trust relationships.
- Seek realistic feedback on your progress through networking, debriefing, and sharing with colleagues (Ares 2018; Baker and Murphy 2021; Faraz 2016; Grosemans et al. 2020; Hussein et al. 2017; Kowalski 2019; Owens 2019; Stewart 2020; Russell and Juliff 2021).

Getting Yourself Ready for Your First Job

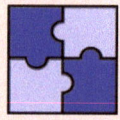

Forethought and reflective journaling have been used throughout this book to help you gain insight into your strengths and your core beliefs of your self-concept and professional identity formation. It can be helpful to prepare yourself for your first job through the review, consideration, and answering the following series of questions (adapted from Baker and Murphy 2021).

1. Did I gain the knowledge about the APN role and scope of practice during my graduate education that I set out to learn? _____

2. What skills and knowledge will I transfer to my new APN role? _____
   _____
   _____

3. When I look back at my graduate education, what am I proudest about? _____
   _____
   _____
   _____

4. How much responsibility and autonomy do I want in my APN job? _____
   _____
   _____
   _____

5. What kind of people do I want to work with? _____
   _____
   _____
   _____

6. What do I seek in my work–life balance? _____
   _____
   _____

7. What are the three most important attributes that I want in my new position? _____
   _____
   _____
   _____

8. What does success look like in 1–2 years? _____
   _____
   _____
   _____

7.6.4   Addition to Your Personal Transition Plan

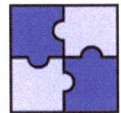

Imposter phenomenon is a real possibility for any person going through a significant role transition. The most effective way to decrease the negative impact to your self-concept and professional identity is early recognition of IP and a pre-designed plan for you to overcome this barrier. Review the information on IP and write a SMART action plan concerning the activities and support you will utilize if these negative thoughts occur during your first several months of APN clinical practice.

Activity   Your Personal Role Transition Plan

Goal: Early recognition of imposter syndrome.
SMART Action Plan. (Specific, measurable, attainable, realistic, time-bond)
I will…….

_____
_____
_____
_____
_____
_____
_____
_____
_____
_____
_____

7.6.5   Tracking Your Transition into the Workplace

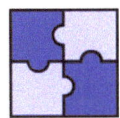

You can use the following "month calendar" to check your role transition to clinical practice progress and to celebrate your success. Month 1 is when you start your new job.
After graduation—before work

7.6.6   Laying the Foundation

1. List one way you relaxed after graduation:

2. Explain why you choose your first job and your anticipation to working there:

3. Who are you support people outside of nursing? Have you shared with them the anticipated next 12 months of role transition? Will you tell them?

The Doing stage	Launching your career		
Month 1	**Month 2**	**Month 3**	**Month 4**
Describe your first day: _____	Describe a diagnosis you made and how you felt about the process?	Describe a good encounter with a peer and the outcomes.	Describe one of your complex patients and how you helped them.
Was the last day of the first month better?	Explain something new you learned?	How are you adjusting to your clinical practice?	Are your skills improving?
Acknowledge your increased understanding of your clinical practice and the people who work there.	Any signs of IP? If yes, what is your plan?		Are you concealing anything?
			Any signs of IP? If yes, what is your plan?

Notes:

_____
_____
_____
_____
_____
_____
_____
_____

The being stage		Meeting the Challenge	
Month 5	**Month 6**	**Month 7**	**Month 8**
How are you meeting the challenges—describe one of your success in month 5.	Review your development of critical think. Explain how that has changed:	Review your personalized competency domain and share your positive outcomes.	Share the development of a trust relationship with someone in your clinical practice or stakeholder.

The being stage		Meeting the Challenge	
Month 5	Month 6	Month 7	Month 8
	Do you have doubts about yourself, your role, or your workplace? If so describe them and make a SMART plan to overcome your doubts.		

Notes:

_____

_____

_____

_____

_____

The Knowing stage		Broadening the perspective	
Month 9	Month 10	Month 11	Month 12
Write about a new responsibility place upon you, or you accepted and your reaction:	How has your time management changed over the last months?

How is your self-concept? | Review your professional identity and write how it has changed with your clinical practice experiences? | Write one SMART action plan on how you plan to help your clinic improve in how they provide care to your community. |

Notes:

_____

_____

_____

_____

_____

_____

_____

_____

_____

7.7 Summary

This last chapter provides an infrastructure to recognize the components of clinical expertise: The APN competency domains. The four integrated domains are intrapersonal and interpersonal relationships, knowledge and skills, creative and critical thinking, and clinical expertise. Each domain is explored to illustrate how the APN role and professional identity formation are integrated in role transition. As knowledge and skills advance through research and technology so will the professional identity change to reflect new wisdom.

Your APN role transition through your graduate education is not your only transition. The second APN transition from the APN graduation to clinical practice can be challenging. Both barriers and facilitators are discussed to provide insight and activities to help build skills for a positive transition into the workplace. Two perspectives of the role transition process are explored: the process of self-awareness with the theory of Limbo to Legitimacy and using time in practice for anticipated achievements and role transition. Although the post-graduation process of role transition can be challenging, several facilitators and activities are provided to aid the APN student prepare for their first APN job and role transition.

References

Ackerman CE (2020) What is self-concept? A psychologist explains. https://positivepsychology.com/self-concept/. Accessed 13 May 2020

Anderson H, Birks Y, Adamson J (2020) Exploring the relationship between nursing identity and advanced nursing practice: an ethnographic study. J Clin Nurs 29:1195–1208. https://doi.org/10.1111/jocn.15155

Ares TL (2018) Role transition after clinical nurse specialist education. Clin Nurse Spec 32(2):71–80. https://doi.org/10.1097/NUR.0000000000000357

Bacal R (n.d.) Leadership development for informal leaders. In: Leadership today. http://leadertoday.org/articles/developinformalleaders.htm. Accessed 4 Feb 2020

Baker EL, Murphy SA (2021) A systematic approach to job transitions—finding your way and landing in the best place. J Public Health Manag Pract 27(1):88–91. https://doi.org/10.1097/PHH.0000000000001231

Bandura A (2018) Toward a psychology of human agency: pathways and reflections. Perspect Psychol Sci 13(2):130–136. https://doi.org/10.1177/1745691617699280

Barlow NA, Hargreaves J, Gillibrand W (2018) Nurses' contributions to the resolution of ethical dilemmas in practice. Nurs Ethics 25(2):230–242. https://doi.org/10.1177/0969733017703700

Barone MA, Vercio C, Jirasevijinda T (2019) Supporting the development of professional identity in the millennial learner. Pediatrics 143(3):e20183988

Beaty RE, Benedek M, Silvia PJ, Schacter DL (2016) Creative cognition and brain network dynamics. Trends Cogn Sci 20(2):87–95. https://doi.org/10.1016/j.tics.2015.10.004

Branch W, George M (2017) Reflection-based learning for professional ethical formation. Am Med Assoc 19(4):349–356

Brown M, Olshansky E (1997) From limbo to legitimacy: a theoretical model of the transition to the primary care nurse practitioner role. Nurs Res 46(1):46–51

Candy PC (1982) Personal constructs and personal paradigms: elaboration, modification, and transformation. Interchange 13:56–69. https://doi.org/10.1007/BF01191423

Chambers M (2018) Interpersonal relationships and communication as a gateway to patient and public involvement and engagement. Health Expect 21(2):407–408. https://doi.org/10.1111/hex.12683

del Mar Molero Jurado M, del Carmen Pérez-Fuentes M, Ruiz NFO, del Mar Simón Márquez M, Linares JJG (2019) Self-efficacy and emotional intelligence as predictors of perceived stress in nursing professionals. Medicina 55:237. https://doi.org/10.3390/medicina55060237

Deliktas A, Korukcu O, Aydin R, Kabukcuoglu K (2019) A nursing students' perceptions of nursing metaparadigms: A phenomenological study. The Journal of Nursing Research 27;5:1–9

Dickert N, Kass N (2009) Understanding respect: learning from patients. J Med Ethics 35(7):419–423. https://doi.org/10.1136/jme.2008.027235

Duchscher JB (2008) A process of becoming: the stages of new nursing graduate professional role transition. J Contin Educ Nurs 39(10):441–450

Dumphy D, DeSandre C, Thompson J (2019) Family nurse practitioner students' perceptions of readiness and transition into advanced practice. Nurs Forum 54:352–357. https://doi.org/10.1111/nuf.12336

Ewertsson M, Bagga-Gutpa S, Alliv R, Bloomberg K (2017) Tensions in learning professional identities—nursing students' narrative and participation in practical skill during clinical practice: an ethnographic study. BMC Nurs 16:48. https://doi.org/10.1186/s12912-017-0238-y

Faraz A (2016) Novice nurse practitioner workforce transition into primary care: a literature review. West J Nurs Res 38(1):1531–1545. https://doi.org/10.1177/0193945916649587

Goliroshan S, Nobahar M, Raeisdana N, Ebadinejad Z, Azizneja droshan P (2021) The protective role of professional self-concept and job embeddedness on nurses' burnout: structural equation modeling. BMC Nurs 20:203. https://doi.org/10.1186/s12912-021-00727-8

Gottlieb M, Chung A, Battaglioli N, Sebok-Syer SS, Kalantari A (2020) Impostor syndrome among physicians and physicians in training: a scoping review. Med Educ 54(2):116–124. https://doi.org/10.1111/medu.13956. Epub 2019 Nov 6. PMID: 31692028

Graf AC, Jacob E, Twigg D, Nattabi B (2020) Contemporary nursing graduates' transition to practice: a critical review of transition models. J Clin Nurs 29(15–16):3097–3107. https://doi.org/10.1111/jocn.15234. Epub 2020 Mar 12. PMID: 32129522

Grosemans I, Coertjens L, Kyndt E (2020) Work-related learning in the transition from high education to work: the role of the development of self-efficacy and achievement goals. Br J Educ Psychol 90:19–42. https://doi.org/10.1111/blep.12258

Hayes MM, Chatterjee S, Schwartzstein RM (2017) Critical thinking in critical care: five strategies to improve teaching and learning in the intensive care unit. Ann Am Thorac Soc 14(4):569–575. https://doi.org/10.1513/AnnalsATS.201612-1009AS

Heitz LJ, Steiner SH, Burman ME (2004) RN to FNP: a qualitative study of role transition. J Nurs Educ 43:416–420

Hussein R, Everett B, Ramjan L, Hu W, Salamonson Y (2017) New graduate nurses' experiences in a clinical speciality: a follow up study of newcomer perceptions of transitional support. BMC Nurs 16:42. https://doi.org/10.1186/s12912-017-0236-0

Ibrahim NK, Algethmi WA, Binshihon SM, Almahyawi RA, Alahmadi RF, Baabdullah MY (2017) Predictors and correlations of emotional intelligence among medical students at King Abdulaziz University, Jeddah. Pak J Med Sci 33(5):1080–1085. https://doi.org/10.12669/pjms.335.13157

Johnson M, Cowin LS, Wilson I, Young H (2012) Professional identity and nursing: contemporary theoretical developments and future research challenges. Int Nurs Rev 59(11):562–569. https://doi.org/10.1111/j.1466-7657.2012.01013.x

Katz H (2018) Informal leadership: leading without authority. https://medium.com/@harry_katz/informal-leadership-leading-without-authority-6373ff4e0a51. (Updated 9 Sept). Accessed 4 Feb 2020

Kidner M (2019) APN role transition with LEAP leadership. Copyright of unpublished works. TXu 2-166-138. The United States Copyright Office

Koloroutis M, Wessler. (2007) Leading empowered organizations. Creative Health Care Management, Minneapolis

Kowalski K (2019) Mentoring. J Contin Educ Nurs 50(12):540–541. https://doi.org/10.3928/00220124-20191115-04

Millick C (2012) Values-based leadership and happiness: enlightened leadership improves the return on people. The Journal of Values-Based Leadership 2(2)Article 5

Mullangi S, Jagsi R (2019) Imposter syndrome: treat the cause, not the symptom. JAMA 322(5):403–404. https://doi.org/10.1001/jama.2019.9788. PMID: 31386138

Oleś PK, Brinthaupt TM, Dier R, Polak D (2020) Types of inner dialogues and functions of self-talk: comparisons and implications. Front Psychol 11:227. Published 2020 Mar 6. https://doi.org/10.3389/fpsyg.2020.00227

Owens R (2019) Nurse practitioner role transition and identity development in rural health care settings: a scoping review. Nurs Educ Perspect 40(3):157–161. https://doi.org/10.1097/01.NEP.0000000000000455

Parschau L et al (2013) Positive experience, self-efficacy, and action control predict physical activity changes: a moderate mediation analysis. Br J Health Psychol 18:395–406. https://doi.org/10.1111/j.2044-8287.2012.02099.x

Poronsky CB (2013) Exploring the transition from registered nurse to family nurse practitioner. J Prof Nurs 29(6):350–358. https://doi.org/10.1016/j.profnurs.2012.10.011

Purc E, Laguna M (2019) Personal values and innovative behavior of employees. Front Psychol 2019(10):865. https://doi.org/10.3389/fpsyg.2019.00865

Roberto MA (2011) Transformational leadership: How leaders change ream, companies, and organizations. The Great Courses. Chantilly, Virginia

Russell K, Juliff D (2021) Graduate nurse transition programs pivotal point of participant' practice readiness questioned during the Covid-19 pandemic crisis: a scoping review. J Contin Educ Nurs 52(8):392–396. https://doi.org/10.3928/00220124-20210714-09

Scott KT (2009) The integrated work of leadership: a journey of transformation. Ki ThoughtBridge LLC, Indianapolis

Sinusoid D (2021) Are your personal paradigms truly your own? https://www.shortform.com/blog/personal-paradigm/. Accessed 25 Apr 2022

Stewart D (n.d.) Mentorship. Conference presentation at fellows of the American Association of Nurse Practitioners Winter Meeting, 2020 Feb. 29; Austin, Texas

Thompson A (2019) An educational intervention to enhance nurse practitioner role transition in the first year of practice. Am Assoc Nurse Pract 31(1):24–32. https://doi.org/10.1097/jxx.0000000000000095

Trede F (2012) Role of work-integrated learning in developing professionalism and professional identity. Asia Pac J Coop Educ 13(3):159–167

Trede F, Macklin R, Bridges D (2011) Professional identity development: a review of the higher education literature. Stud High Educ 37(3):365–384. https://doi.org/10.1080/03075079.2010.521237

Vaismoradi M, Salsali M, Ahmadi F (2011) Perspective of Iranian male nursing students regarding the role of nursing education in developing a professional-identity: a content analysis study. Jpn J Nurs Sci 8:174–183. https://doi.org/10.1111/j.1742-7924.2010.00172.x

Von Collin-Appling C, Giuliano D (2017) A concept analysis of critical thinking: a guide for nurse educators. Nurse Educ Today 49:106–109. https://doi.org/10.1016/j.nedt.2016.11.007